MIDTown VET

W9-BHA-972

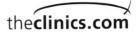

VETERINARY CLINICS

CLINICS

OF NORTH AMERICA

Small Animal Practice

Practice Management

GUEST EDITOR
David E. Lee, DVM, MBA

March 2006 • Volume 36 • Number 2

SAUNDERS

An Imprint of Elsevier, Inc.
PHILADELPHIA   LONDON   TORONTO   MONTREAL   SYDNEY   TOKYO

W.B. SAUNDERS COMPANY
A Division of Elsevier Inc.

Elsevier, Inc., 1600 John F. Kennedy Blvd., Suite 1800, Philadelphia, PA 19103-2899

http://www.vetsmall.theclinics.com

VETERINARY CLINICS OF NORTH AMERICA:	**Volume 36, Number 2**
SMALL ANIMAL PRACTICE	**ISSN 0195-5616**
March 2006	**ISBN 1-4160-3582-6**
Editor: John Vassallo	

Veterinary Clinics of North America: Small Animal Practice (ISSN 0195-5616) is published bimonthly (For Post Office use only: volume 36 issue 2 of 6) by Elsevier, Inc. Corporate and editorial offices: Elsevier, Inc., 1600 John F. Kennedy Blvd., Suite 1800, Philadelphia, PA 19103-2899. Accounting and circulation offices: 6277 Sea Harbor Drive, Orlando, FL 32887-4800. Periodicals postage paid at Orlando, FL 32862, and additional mailing offices. Subscription prices are $170.00 per year for US individuals, $275.00 per year for US institutions, $85.00 per year for US students and residents, $225.00 per year for Canadian individuals, $345.00 per year for Canadian institutions, $235.00 per year for international individuals, $345.00 per year for international institutions and $115.00 per year for Canadian and foreign students/residents. To receive student/resident rate, orders must be accompanied by name of affiliated institution, date of term, and the *signature* of program/residency coordinator on institution letterhead. Orders will be billed at individual rate until proof of status is received. Foreign air speed delivery is included in all *Clinics* subscription prices. All prices are subject to change without notice. POSTMASTER: Send address changes to *Veterinary Clinics of North America: Small Animal Practice*, Elsevier, Customer Service Department, 6277 Sea Harbor Drive, Orlando, FL 32887-4800, USA; phone: (+1)(877) 839-7126 [toll free number for US customers], or (+1)(407) 345-4020 [customers outside US]; fax: (+1)(407) 363-1354; email: usjcs@elsevier.com.

Veterinary Clinics of North America: Small Animal Practice is also published in Japanese by Gakusosha Company Ltd., 2-16-28 Nishikata, Bunkyo-ku, Tokyo 113, Japan.

Reprints: For copies of 100 or more, of articles in this publication, please contact the Commercial Reprints Department, Elsevier Inc., 360 Park Avenue South, New York, New York 10010-1710. Tel. (212) 633-3813 Fax: (212) 462-1935, email: reprints@elsevier.com

Veterinary Clinics of North America: Small Animal Practice is covered in *Current Contents/Agriculture, Biology and Environmental Sciences, Science Citation Index, ASCA, Index Medicus, Excerpta Medica,* and *BIOSIS.*

Printed in the United States of America.

VETERINARY CLINICS
SMALL ANIMAL PRACTICE

Practice Management

GUEST EDITOR

DAVID E. LEE, DVM, MBA, Hospital Director and Associate Professor, Practice Management, Veterinary Medical Center, Colorado State University, Fort Collins, Colorado

CONTRIBUTORS

THOMAS E. CATANZARO, DVM, MHA, FACHE, Diplomate, American College of Healthcare Executives; President/CEO, Veterinary Practice Consultants, Golden, Colorado

LOUISE DUNN, Snowgoose Veterinary Management Consulting, Greensboro, North Carolina

MARSHA L. HEINKE, DVM, EA, CPA, CVPM, President and Chief Executive Officer, Marsha L. Heinke, CPA, Inc., Grafton, Ohio

CHARLOTTE A. LACROIX, DVM, JD, Chief Executive Officer of Veterinary Business Advisors, Inc., Whitehouse Station, New Jersey; Adjunct Professor, University of Pennsylvania School of Veterinary Medicine, Philadelphia, Pennsylvania

DAVID E. LEE, DVM, MBA, Hospital Director and Associate Professor, Practice Management, Veterinary Medical Center, Colorado State University, Fort Collins, Colorado

LORRAINE MONHEISER LIST, CPA, MEd, Summit Veterinary Advisors, LLC, Littleton, Colorado

JAMES W. LLOYD, DVM, PhD, Professor, Assistant to the Dean, and Director, Office of Strategy and Innovation, College of Veterinary Medicine, Michigan State University, East Lansing, Michigan

LARRY F. McCORMICK, DVM, MBA, Certified Business Appraiser, Simmons and Associates Mid-Atlantic, Boalsburg, Pennsylvania

THOMAS McFERSON, CPA, ABV, Accredited Business Valuations, Gatto McFerson, CPAs, Santa Monica, California

KARL R. SALZSIEDER, DVM, JD, Salzsieder Consulting and Legal Services, Kelso, Washington

JANE R. SHAW, DVM, PhD, Assistant Professor of Veterinary Communication and Director, Argus Institute, Department of Clinical Sciences, College of Veterinary Medicine and Biomedical Sciences, Colorado State University, Fort Collins, Colorado

CARIN A. SMITH, DVM, Smith Veterinary Consulting, Peshastin, Washington

BONITA S. VOILAND, MS, Assistant Dean for Hospital Operations, Cornell University Hospital for Animals, College of Veterinary Medicine, Ithaca, New York

CHARLES J. WAYNER, DVM, Director, Global Veterinary Practice Health[SM], Hill's Pet Nutrition, Inc., Topeka, Kansas

VETERINARY CLINICS
SMALL ANIMAL PRACTICE

Practice Management

CONTENTS

VOLUME 36 • NUMBER 2 • MARCH 2006

This article explores the economic trends affecting the future of the veterinary medical profession. Key aspects of demand and supply are considered, as are several broad-based institutional factors. Demand for veterinarians and veterinary medical services is demonstrating a definitive upward trend across the profession, led by a remarkable increase in consumers' willingness to spend on animal health care. Supply is also expanding through increased enrollments at colleges and schools of veterinary medicine and increased productivity and efficiency in private practice. Veterinarians' incomes are increasing, and some sectors of the profession offer outstanding financial opportunities. Provided that critical needs are met for 1) increased diversity and 2) continued improvement in the nontechnical capabilites of veterinarians, the outlook for the economic future of the veterinary medical profession is strong.

Marketing is a holistic process that goes far beyond a Yellow Page advertisement or a glossy brochure. A thorough evaluation of a market before entry, including best and worst case scenarios, is critical to making good investments. Veterinarians are fortunate to have a market that is largely protected by barriers to entry and characterized by reasonably high rates of return given minimal risk. Our market base continues to expand and, overall, remains fairly price insensitive. The extent to which a practice can align its capabilities with a product mix that ideally meets its clients' needs will ultimately determine its success.

This article comprises discussions on practices with little or no salable value, the determination and measurement of the value of a veterinary practice, the evolution of the small animal practice marketplace, the costs of selling a portion of a practice, lack of marketability discount, and C corporation issues.

The gender shift in veterinary medicine has paralleled other changes in debt and income. Cause and effect are complex and often confused. Popular notions of the priorities of the new generation of men and women are often not supported by research studies. Recent data reveal new insights into questions surrounding the gender issue.

In the last decade, the veterinary profession has experienced many changes, including the birth of a new area of law known as "animal law," and an increased scrutiny by the legal community and veterinary state boards. This article provides a sampling of some of the more challenging issues the profession is facing in the early part of the 21st century, namely, guardianship versus ownership, the awarding of non-economic damages in negligence lawsuits, and challenges in maintaining medical records.

This article provides the reader with an appreciation of the diverse elements that go into a buy-sell, affiliation, or merger situation for veterinary practices. In the changing market place of American veterinary medicine, old paradigms no longer hold comfort. The generational differences are briefly explored herein as well as the new economic realities. A few examples are offered to illustrate just how much variability exists in the current business of veterinary medicine and the subsequent practice transitions needed to enhance value. Functioning models are explored, as well as affiliation and merger options. Practice valuation is discussed in general terms, referencing the cutting-edge factors. The six-point summary provides almost all practices a solid operational base for daily operations and succession planning.

The major factors to be considered in the real estate purchase decision are the interest rate, the depreciation schedule, the property appreciation, the income tax impact, and the impact of paying a principal payment as part of the real estate mortgage. All these factors must be compared with the costs of leasing.

For 40 years, medical researchers have been studying physician-patient interactions, and the results of these studies have yielded three basic conclusions: physician-patient interactions have an impact on patient health, patient and physician satisfaction, adherence to medical recommendations, and malpractice risk; communication is a core clinical skill and an essential component of clinical competence; and appropriate training programs can significantly change medical practitioners' communication knowledge, skills, and attitudes. Many of these findings are applicable to the practice of veterinary medicine.

Like preparing for intricate surgery, successful staffing requires preparation, mastery of the subject matter, and skill. The employees who work in veterinary practices form the basis of the business and reflect the owners' own values. Giving attention to what you want your practice to be, whom you want working with you, and how the environment keeps the staff productive matters. Identifying the right culture, hiring people who find congruence with the practice's culture, and consistently applying these principles will help your practice soar to new heights.

Rising veterinary costs can keep some people from accepting necessary medical care for their pets. This article discusses viable alternative financing options. Each alternative comes with its own pros and cons. Practice owners will want to study the offerings carefully to find the best match for their practice and clients.

The concept of compliance involves the consistency and accuracy with which a client follows the regimen recommended by the veterinarian or other veterinary health care team member. Contrary to common belief, most compliance failures are not the direct result of a client's unwillingness to comply. This article will help the reader better appreciate the critical importance of effective communication by the entire veterinary health care team in achieving compliance. Success is predicated on an alliance between the practice team and the client. Certain paradigms surrounding compliance in veterinary practice are discussed, and the positive outcomes of compliance, including optimal patient care, exceptional client service, employee career growth, and economic ramifications, are explored.

GOAL STATEMENT

The goal of the *Veterinary Clinics of North America: Small Animal Practice* is to keep practicing veterinarians up to date with current clinical practice in small animal medicine by providing timely articles reviewing the state of the art in small animal care.

ACCREDITATION

The *Veterinary Clinics of North America: Small Animal Practice* offers continuing education credits, awarded by Cummings School of Veterinary Medicine at Tufts University, Office of Continuing Education.

Cummings School of Veterinary Medicine at Tufts University is a designated provider of continuing veterinary medical education. Veterinarians participating in this learning activity may earn up to 6 credits per issue up to a maximum of 36 credits per year. Credits awarded may not apply toward license renewal in all states. It is the responsibility of each participant to verify the requirements of their state licensing board.

Credit can be earned by reading the text material, taking the examination online at ***http:// www.theclinics.com/home/cme***, and completing the program evaluation. Following your completion of the test and program evaluation, and review of any and all incorrect answers, you may print your certificate.

TO ENROLL

To enroll in the *Veterinary Clinics of North America: Small Animal Practice* Continuing Veterinary Medical Education Program, call customer service at 1-800-654-2452 or sign up online at ***http:// www.theclinics.com/home/cme***. The CVME program is now available at a special introductory rate of $99.95 for a year's subscription.

VETERINARY CLINICS
SMALL ANIMAL PRACTICE

ELSEVIER
SAUNDERS

Vet Clin Small Anim 36 (2006) xi–xii

VETERINARY CLINICS
SMALL ANIMAL PRACTICE

PREFACE

Practice Management

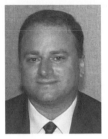

David E. Lee, DVM, MBA

Guest Editor

irst, let me state that I am proud to be a part of a profession filled with individuals who continue to place the welfare of their patients above nearly all else. When I look out at an audience of veterinary students or a group of practitioners, I can be pretty confident that most in the room chose their profession for the right reasons. If I ask such a group how many chose veterinary medicine for the money, the question brings a few chuckles but a hand never goes up. Still, although most of us chose to become veterinarians to help animals and the people who own them, we can only be truly successful in that endeavor if we take steps to ensure a long and sustainable career. The unfortunate individuals who leave the profession because they cannot make their pluses outweigh their minuses must surely feel unfulfilled in their noble aspirations.

Toward that end, practice management and efforts to improve the economic circumstances of veterinarians and the profession are as critical to veterinary medicine as new diagnostic techniques and treatment protocols. I was pleased that *Veterinary Clinics of North America: Small Animal Practice* was so supportive of a proposed issue devoted to practice management because I knew that its reader base represented practitioners with a sincere interest in continuing education and professional development. In almost all cases, good business is good medicine and vice versa.

The last issue of *Veterinary Clinics of North America: Small Animal Practice* dedicated to practice management was published in November 1983. I had actually submitted my draft table of contents to Elsevier before dredging up that issue from the library's archives, but found it very interesting how pertinent some of the topics still are. An article on computers in veterinary practice management,

0195-5616/06/$ – see front matter
doi:10.1016/j.cvsm.2005.11.002

while discussing "floppy drives" and CRTs, accurately predicted the critical role these systems would have in well-managed practices of the future. Deferred compensation plans, pet health insurance, and marketing are still topics of interest and appear in the current issue, albeit, with the advantage of 22 years of evolution and hindsight.

Greater strides have been made in the area of veterinary practice management in the last 5 to 10 years than probably any other time span in our profession. The 1999 KPMG LLP report entitled "The Current and Future Market for Veterinarians and Veterinary Medical Services in the United States" is sometimes referred to as the "Mega Study," presumably because of its depth, breadth, and bulk. Even after 6 years, the dust disturbed because of this landmark study has still not settled. Those who found fault or took issue with the conclusions made in the study will have to concede that, if nothing else, the KPMG study drew attention to the economic problems facing the profession and launched substantive efforts to improve our plight. Most of us in the profession would agree these efforts have been very successful by almost any metric.

I did not want this issue to pick up from where *Veterinary Clinics of North America: Small Animal Practice* left off in 1983, but rather to carry the ball set in motion by the KPMG study. The topics addressed herein begin with a broad overview of current economic trends citing the wealth of information now available to us. Other global issues addressed include a fresh perspective on the cause and effect of the gender shift, as well as current legal issues that impact us all. New associates burdened by significant student loan debt will find the article devoted to buying and selling practices of interest. Buying and leasing real estate for veterinary practice is an area of interest that has received little attention in the past. For current practice owners and administrators, articles on communication, marketing, hiring and retaining excellent employees, billing, third-party payment, and pet health insurance, as well as client compliance, will be pertinent. Practice owners considering a transition into retirement will be particularly interested in the articles on practice valuation and succession planning.

In assembling the team for this project, I had a good idea of which individuals were preeminent in these areas of expertise. I approached them with some trepidation, even the ones whom I knew well, recognizing how busy each of them must be. I had little compensation to offer, only the opportunity to reach a new venue of veterinarians with their critical messages. I was very pleased to discover that the consultants, academicians, and administrators featured herein proved to be every bit as altruistic in their commitment to improving veterinary medicine as the practitioners they serve.

David E. Lee, DVM, MBA
Veterinary Medical Center
Colorado State University
300 W. Drake Road
Fort Collins, CO 80526, USA

E-mail address: dlee@colostate.edu

Vet Clin Small Anim 36 (2006) 267–279

VETERINARY CLINICS
SMALL ANIMAL PRACTICE

Current Economic Trends Affecting the Veterinary Medical Profession

James W. Lloyd, DVM, PhD

Office of Strategy and Innovation, College of Veterinary Medicine, Michigan State University, A110 Veterinary Medical Center, East Lansing, MI 48824, USA

Much has been written in recent years regarding the economics of the veterinary medical profession. Ultimately, the economic health of the veterinary medical profession is closely linked to societal needs for veterinary medical services. To the extent that the veterinary profession effectively meets societal needs, there is a general correlation with willingness to pay for the various services that veterinarians provide. Such willingness to pay, in turn, should provide a sustained economic base from which the veterinary profession can operate and continue to serve society effectively. Such broad statements oversimplify the complex and dynamic economic forces that directly affect veterinary medicine, however. The purpose of this article is to explore some of those forces and their potential implications for the future.

Assessments of the veterinary medical profession's economic health and outlook have historically been neither positive nor optimistic. In an overview of his work published in 1997, Getz [1] made the following assertions: 1. the market for veterinarians is already saturated, 2. career prospects are poor relative to other professions, 3. career prospects will continue to deteriorate, 4. careers in veterinary medicine are unlikely to become more attractive economically over the next decade.

Based on his analysis, Getz [1] predicted that the economic health of the veterinary medical profession would further decline substantially unless the supply of veterinarians could be decreased through scaling back enrollments in the schools and colleges of veterinary medicine. As is shown here, neither the scaling back nor the economic decline has taken place. The economic health of the veterinary profession is much stronger than depicted by Getz [1].

Following the work of Getz [1], the American Veterinary Medical Association (AVMA), the American Animal Hospital Association (AAHA), and the Association of American Veterinary Medical Colleges (AAVMC) joined together to commission a comprehensive study [2] of the veterinary medical

E-mail address: lloydj@cvm.msu.edu

0195-5616/06/$ – see front matter
doi:10.1016/j.cvsm.2005.10.008

profession. The purpose of the study was to ensure that the profession would remain productive, responsive, and economically successful. Conducted by KPMG LLP, the results of this work (commonly known as the Mega Study) also depicted poor economic health in the veterinary profession and suggested an oversupply of veterinarians similar to Getz [1]. The study was a bit more optimistic, however, in that it also documented a noteworthy increase in the demand for veterinary services that was projected to continue into the foreseeable future. One of the primary elements underlying this positive trend in demand was a steady increase in consumers' willingness to pay for veterinary services, which was also projected to carry into the future. Another key finding of the study was that certain nontechnical skills, knowledge, aptitudes, and attitudes (SKAs) of veterinarians may be lacking in the veterinary profession and, thereby, may be limiting the potential economic and professional growth being achieved. In addition, it was suggested that other factors were important to consider when contemplating the future economic health of the veterinary profession, including the gender shift toward an increasing proportion of female veterinarians and inherent inefficiency in traditional animal health care delivery systems.

Soon after the Mega Study was published, another national study [3] concurred with the previous findings that the economic health of the veterinary medical profession (in this case, represented by individual veterinarians' incomes) was being constrained by a lack of certain nontechnical SKAs. In addition, the study noted a substantial difference between the earnings of male and female veterinarians. These findings were supported by yet another more recent study [4] conducted by many of the same investigators.

Collectively, these prior studies provide a sense of the veterinary medical profession's recent economic history. Their findings and recommendations also form an invaluable context for considering the profession's current economic health and potential trends for the future.

MARKET STRUCTURE

Before contemplating the current economic trends of importance to veterinary medicine, it should be useful to review key features of the underlying market structures. Toward that end, it is first appropriate to recognize the key differences between the market for veterinary medical services and the market for veterinarians. The latter is a professional labor market, where the buyers include various organizations that employ veterinarians and the sellers are the veterinarians themselves. Payment in this market takes the form of salaries, wages, and benefits, for example.

In 2005, 78.3% of AVMA members who provided information on their primary employer indicated that they worked in private practice [5]. Because most veterinarians are employed in clinical practice settings, the primary labor market for veterinarians is largely driven by the underlying market for clinical veterinary medical services. This market, in turn, is composed of consumers of veterinary medical services (primarily animal owners) and the organizations that provide these services (veterinary practices). Payment in this particular market takes the form of the various fees for service that characterize veterinary practices.

Economists would describe the market for veterinary medical services as a "monopolistic competition" [6]. In this special type of market characterized by many relatively small firms, the number of buyers far exceeds the number of sellers and the products are differentiated (nonidentical) from seller to seller, although the products of any one seller can serve as strong substitutes for products from other individual sellers. As a result of this differentiation, consumers face numerous choice factors, only one of which is price. In fact, the greater the product differentiation between respective sellers, the less sensitive are consumers to price as a determinant of demand, such that changes in price have a relatively small impact on the quantity of the products purchased (proportionately speaking, as compared with the proportionate change in price). When this reality is embraced by sellers in such markets, firms generally have the opportunity to price their products in a manner that leads to consistently strong demand and an accompanying sustained level of profitability (especially when this occurs in the presence of any substantial entry barriers). These sellers need not behave as price takers. If sellers behave as price takers, competing primarily on the basis of price, profitability is almost certain to be restricted as a consequence.

What this means for veterinarians is that those practices (sellers) that work progressively to differentiate their services from those of other neighboring practices (based on factors like technology, customer service, locations, hours of operation, and SKAs of the attending veterinarians) should expect the opportunity to price their services in a manner that leads to a consistently strong client base and an accompanying sustained profitability. To the extent that these features are embraced across the broad base of the private practice community, the derived demand for veterinarians (labor market) is also expected to be consistently strong, leading to a sustained opportunity for attractive levels of earnings for the veterinarians involved. Because private practice comprises such a large portion of the labor market for veterinarians, it is reasonable to infer that the dynamics of the veterinary services market have a broad impact on veterinary incomes. Consequently, a trend toward conscious progressive differentiation of veterinary services between practices should be expected to have positive economic effects across the profession. This directly implies a critical need for certain SKAs to enable recognition of the opportunities available through differentiation and for practices to achieve the resulting consistent economic success, however.

KEY TRENDS

Based on the preceding discussion, it is clear that the demand for veterinary medical services and the demand for veterinarians are closely linked, although not identical. Similar claims can be made for the supply side of the equation.

For these reasons, demand trends are discussed as a single category, as are supply trends. Subsequently, institutional trends are also considered.

Demand

As previously mentioned, the KPMG study predicted a steady growth in the demand for veterinary medical services led primarily by the demand for companion animal services [2]. As indicated by consumers' increasing willingness to spend on pet health care, pet owners have collectively demonstrated a consistent interest in improving the health and well-being of their companion animals as a key dimension of the evolving nature of the human-animal bond. On a related note, forthcoming research results indicate that the income elasticity of demand for veterinary services is decreasing over time, indicating that the quantity of veterinary services purchased by individual consumers is becoming less and less dependent on those consumers' income levels (C. Wolf, PhD, Department of Agricultural Economics, Michigan State University, East Lansing, Michigan, personal communication, September 2005). In that context, recent research on client compliance [7] with veterinary health care recommendations indicates that the opportunity exists to enhance the quality of health care substantially within the boundaries of existing science and technology, assuming development of effective client education and marketing programs (another SKA issue). In addition to general practice services for companion animals but consistent with the trend in willingness to spend, an increasing demand for specialty-trained veterinarians has also been suggested [8].

To the extent that 94.3% of horse owners responding to a recent survey considered their horse to be a "family member" or "pet/companion" [9], many aspects of equine practice parallel companion animal practice. In this case, demand trends in equine practice can be expected to be somewhat similar to those of companion animal practice. This is particularly true of pleasure horse practice. Some facets of equine practice (especially those that involve certain types of working and competitive animals) are more likely to ebb and flow with local, state, and national economic conditions, however.

For food animal species, trends in demand for veterinarians and veterinary medical services are driven by structural changes in the livestock industry and changes in the demand for livestock products. Widespread consolidation in the livestock industries has markedly changed the types and quantities of veterinary services demanded. The dynamics of demand in this market are currently under extensive study by a group of researchers at Kansas State University, who project modest (<10%) increases in the demand for veterinary services in this sector over the next few years (D. Andrus, PhD; B. Prince, PhD; and K. Gwinner, PhD; Kansas State University, Manhattan, Kansas, personal communication at the AVMA Annual Conference in Minneapolis, July 2005).

A closely related market is that associated with the demand for veterinarians and veterinary medical services in public practice and public health careers. Together with food animal practice, it is estimated that satisfying only current needs in population health and public practice in the United States should require more than 500 of the approximately 2500 available new US graduates each year for the foreseeable future [10]. These needs are driven by several factors, including post-"9/11" concerns related to the potential for bio- and agro-terrorism; the high proportion of emerging and re-emerging infectious diseases that are zoonotic; continued consumer trends expanding interest in food safety; and the skewed age distribution of incumbents holding such positions, which portends a potentially crippling wave of impending retirements.

This picture gains an added dimension when the potential impact of international livestock markets is considered. A study conducted in the late 1990s describes a "revolution" in global agriculture, whereby the global demand for livestock products is predicted to nearly double during the first 20 years of the twenty-first century [11]. Although the specific impact that this revolution may have on the global or US demand for veterinary services is not discussed, the presence of twice as much livestock on the globe can certainly be expected to have a substantial impact of some sort. Because the report predicts that the greatest expansion of livestock production is likely to occur in developing countries, it might reasonably be expected that the biggest impact on veterinary medicine would be internationally in the government and industry employment sectors, because private practice has not been consistently successful in these countries (as a general rule).

For the most part, trends in the demand for veterinarians in industry can be expected to follow the broader professional trends discussed within the other sectors, with the possible exception of research. A recent report by the National Academy of Sciences [12] recommends expanding the veterinary research work force to achieve critical enduring advances in animal and human health. Based on current patterns, the distribution of this expansion would be expected to encompass industry, government (addressed previously), and academia.

An increased number of veterinary medical researchers in the academic sector would augment the suggested need for additional clinical faculty (R. Richardson, DVM, Dean, College of Veterinary Medicine, Kansas State University, Manhattan, Kansas, personal communication at the AAVMC Annual Conference in Washington, DC, March 2005). An expansion of clinical faculty would be allocated to roles of teaching (veterinary students, interns, and residents), clinical service, and clinical research.

Supply

The primary influence on the supply of veterinarians and veterinary medical services is the entry of new veterinarians into the profession. With the main source of these entrants being graduation from the colleges and schools of veterinary medicine, it is insightful to consider enrollment trends across the AAVMC [13], for which data are presented in Table 1. Over the past 6 years, graduations from US and Canadian colleges and schools of veterinary medicine (approximated by year 4 enrollments) have increased by 2.2%. During the same period, admissions to these institutions (approximated by year 1 enrollments) have increased by 8.5%. Of this 8.5% increase, approximately 3.0%

Table 1
Veterinary student enrollments by year, Association of American Veterinary Medical Colleges member institutions, 1999–2000 through 2004–2005

Report year	Year 1	Year 2	Year 3	Year 4	Grand total
1999–2000	2674	2609	2523	2537	10,343
2000–2001	2696	2648	2570	2509	10,423
2001–2002	2700	2644	2321	2567	10,532
2002–2003	2655	2590	2545	2548	10,338
2003–2004	2825	2642	2567	2550	10,584
2004–2005	2901	2843	2682	2594	11,020

Data from Association of American Veterinary Medical Colleges. Comparative data reports, 1999–2000 through 2004–2005. Washington (DC): Association of American Veterinary Medical Colleges; 2000–2005.

can be attributed to the addition of one new school [13]. The remaining 5.5% is apparently associated with increasing class sizes among the existing colleges and schools, however. Although supporting data were not readily available, anecdotal evidence suggests that the North American colleges and schools of veterinary medicine outside the United States and Canada may be expanding enrollment at an even greater rate than the US and Canadian institutions.

Because the number of veterinarians is expected to increase, the demographics of the population of veterinarians become of interest. The KPMG study analyzed the gender shift that is underway in the veterinary profession and predicted that female veterinarians would outnumber male veterinarians after the year 2004 and that the percentage of women in the profession would reach 67% by 2015 [2]. As of December 31, 2004, the gender breakdown of AVMA members who were actively employed was 54% male and 46% female (A. Shepherd, MBA, Research Projects Manager, Communications Division, AVMA, Schaumburg, Illinois, personal communication, September 6, 2005). Although it seems that the trend has not quite fulfilled the KPMG predictions at this point, the overall pattern is not substantially different from that foreseen by the study.

Other demographic dimensions are also critical to consider as indicators of the degree of diversity inherent in the population of veterinarians. Best estimates indicate that the proportion of underrepresented minorities entering the profession has increased from 4.1% in 1981 to 9.7% in 2005 [14]. Although data on race and ethnicity do not currently exist for the veterinary profession as a whole, the actual proportion of nonwhite veterinarians in the profession would be expected to be considerably less than 10% based on the enrollment trend and expected attrition (in veterinary school and after graduation). Data on sexual orientation, disabilities, and other key diversity indicators are not readily available for the veterinary profession.

Beyond demographics, the prevalence and distribution of additional characteristics are important to consider when contemplating the supply of veterinarians. Consistent with the associated increasing demand (previously mentioned), the AVMA reports 7970 specialty-trained veterinarians [15]. Although probably not all these specialists are AVMA members, and perhaps not all are active, the number is equivalent to 11.2% of the total AVMA membership and 12.3% of total active veterinarians [5]. For the most part, these veterinarians are employed by academic institutions and an increasing number of private specialty practices. In 2005, approximately 19% of all AAVMC graduates (498 of 2594 individuals) pursued advanced clinical training in the form of an internship recognized and matched by the American Association of Veterinary Clinicians (AAVC) (M. Garvey, DVM, Animal Medical Center, New York, New York, personal communication at the AAVC Annual Conference in Atlanta, March 2005) [13]. Of these, approximately 46% (217 of 477 graduates) go on to pursue specialty training in the form of AAVC-recognized (and matched) residency positions. (These numbers should be viewed as approximations in that the AAVMC number is actually year 4 enrollments and the AAVC numbers include an unknown number of foreign graduates.) Although trend data on these numbers are not available, it can be seen that specialty training is a substantial factor when considering the supply of veterinarians and veterinary services.

In addition to clinical skills, current trends indicate that the nontechnical SKAs of veterinarians should continue to improve in the future. In response to the challenge posed by the KPMG study results, at least 23 of 27 US colleges and schools of veterinary medicine had implemented some sort of programmatic change by 2003 with the intent of enhancing students' SKAs [16]. Unpublished data indicate that the response had reached 29 of 31 AAVMC members by early 2005. These programmatic changes were found to be generally consistent with the specific recommendations offered by studies focused on the applicant pool [17], admissions [18], curriculum (and cocurricular experiences) [19], veterinary teaching hospital [20], and leadership needs in veterinary medicine [21]. Ongoing SKA dialogue across the AAVMC and within many individual colleges and schools of veterinary medicine (H. Rubin, MBA, CEO, National Commission on Veterinary Economic Issues, Schaumburg, Illinois, personal communication, July 2005) provides anecdotal evidence suggesting that this trend is likely to continue.

From an economic perspective, the key factors to consider in characterizing the supply side of any market include price and cost structures. With regard to the supply of veterinarians, these factors are reflected by veterinary incomes and average debt load of new graduates, respectively. The most recent data available from the AVMA indicate that the average veterinarian earned $101,040 in private practice and $103,750 in public or corporate practice during 2003 [22]. Since 1995, these incomes have increased by 75.7% in nominal terms (no adjustment for inflation) and by 37.6% in real terms (adjusted for inflation) [23]. These numbers represent an average annual nominal increase of 9.5% and an average annual real increase of 4.7% over the 8-year period. Although the increases have not been as rapid, salaries of new graduates have followed a similar trend. The average income of new graduates entering private practice in 2004 was \$49,635 [24], which showed a nominal increase since 1999 of 28.8% and a real increase of 13.6% [25]. On an average annual basis over this 5-year period, these increases are approximately 5.8% (nominal) and 2.7% (real).

Recent data from the AVMA also indicate that 88.2% of new graduates in 2004 were carrying educational debt at time of graduation, and this debt averaged \$81,052 for these individuals [24]. This finding is consistent with an upward trend in debt load among new graduates, which has increased by 28.5% (nominal) and by 13.3% (real) since 1999 [25]. On an average annual basis, these increases in debt load are approximately 5.7% (nominal) and 2.7% (real) over the 5-year period.

From a broad perspective, it is also evident that substantial structural change is underway on the supply side of the market for veterinary medical services. Together, these ongoing changes ultimately stem from changes in available technology and the evolution of demand; cost structures, efficiencies, and profitabilities can be expected to change as a result.

Two key trends that point to the existence of structural change relate to practice size and the ratio of nonveterinarians to veterinarians. Table 2 contains AVMA data from 1995 and 2003 pertaining to staffing levels for the six primary types of private veterinary practice. Without exception, it can be seen from these data that practice size (as indicated by the number of full-time-equivalent [FTE] veterinarians per practice) increased over the 8-year period. In addition, the ratio of staff to veterinarians has increased for every type of practice except "Large Animal Exclusive," which is basically unchanged. Although tests of statistical significance are not available to establish definitive confidence in the apparent difference between means, the remarkable consistency of the pattern that is evident across practice types is compelling evidence for the existence of a real trend. Evolution of these staffing patterns in the provision of veterinary services should undoubtedly influence and improve the

Table 2
Practice size and ratio of staff to veterinarians (full-time-equivalent basis), American Veterinary Medical Association, 1995 and 2003

Practice type	1995			2003		
	Staff	Veterinarians	Ratio	Staff	Veterinarians	Ratio
Large animal exclusive	2.15	2.03	1.06	3.30	3.25	1.02
Large animal predominant	2.82	2.53	1.11	4.20	2.77	1.52
Mixed	4.46	2.43	1.84	5.90	2.91	2.03
Small animal predominant	4.56	2.01	2.27	7.50	2.18	3.44
Small animal exclusive	5.03	1.82	2.76	8.10	2.25	3.60
Equine	2.21	1.65	1.34	4.00	2.83	1.41

Data from American Veterinary Medical Association. Economic report on veterinarians and veterinary practices: 2005 edition. Schaumburg (IL): American Veterinary Medical Association; 2005; and American Veterinary Medical Association. Economic report on veterinarians and veterinary practices. Schaumburg (IL): American Veterinary Medical Association; 1997.

efficiency of operations and, consequently, tend to improve cost structures within the private practice sector.

Additional structural change is underway with regard to science and technology. With its base in the medical sciences, continual advances in science and technology directly affect veterinary medicine through the accompanying rapid progression of available services and approaches to health management. As science and technology continue to advance, the level of sophistication that is feasible in animal health management should advance in step. As a consequence, cost structures can again be expected to change, although the net impact on efficiencies is unclear. Some advances in technology can be expected to improve efficiencies markedly through decreasing the amount of time required for certain procedures, decreasing the need for other complementary inputs (eg, certain medical supplies, aftercare), or improving outcomes. Advanced technology can often be expensive, however, and the associated capital investment can potentially have a negative impact on efficiencies, depending on the relative level of demand and the appropriateness of accompanying pricing decisions.

The rising costs of human health care are also affecting structural change across the veterinary medical profession. Driven by science, technology, and the legal environment, the relentless increase in the cost of medical insurance is having an adverse effect on the cost of human resources in virtually every sector of the veterinary profession. The ability to recruit and retain the right people for the job is key to the success of any organization [26]. Being able to offer health insurance benefits as part of a compensation package can be vital to hiring and retaining the right people but is becoming increasingly costly.

One sector of the veterinary medical profession that has not escaped the rising costs of human health care and medical insurance or the rising costs of cutting-edge medial technology is academic veterinary medicine. Although these operating costs have been escalating for academic institutions, a substantial negative trend in the level of governmental support for higher education has developed over the same period. The resulting upward pressure on the costs of training veterinary students has been considerable, and tuition costs for veterinary students have necessarily increased as a consequence. This situation helps to explain the previously mentioned upward trend in new graduate debt loads and serves to place considerable upward pressure on the salaries of new graduates. Although the increasing salaries have seemingly kept pace with the increasing debt loads (as discussed), the impact on employers across all sectors of the market for veterinary services is that another dimension of the cost structure is drifting upward.

Institutional

The final category of trends to be considered is referred to as institutional because it contains factors that are broad based or societal, often affecting supply and demand. Several such broad-based trends have already been briefly mentioned in previous sections as they more directly affect the supply or demand for veterinarians or veterinary services. Those previously discussed include trends related to food safety, post-9/11 concerns for bio- and agroterrorism, zo-onotic emerging and re-emerging infectious diseases, the human-animal bond, trends in science and technology, expanding costs of human health care, and shifts in the patterns of funding for higher education. Other such trends with a more general impact are addressed at this point.

To discuss economic trends of importance to the veterinary medical profession without including mention of such universally important issues as interest rates, inflation rates, unemployment rates, and economic growth would be an egregious oversight. These factors are ubiquitous in their economic importance, and veterinary medicine offers no exception. For the most part, the impact of these factors on the markets for veterinarians and veterinary services tend to mirror the impact on the economy as a whole; thus, further consideration beyond those aspects already considered is probably not warranted.

Other broad-based trends can be expected to have a much more specific impact on the veterinary medical profession, however. One such trend involves the demographic characteristics of the consuming public. As previously mentioned, the proportion of underrepresented minorities in the AVMA membership is estimated be less than 10% based on the demographics of AAVMC student enrollments [14]. This compares to an estimate from the US Census Bureau indicating that the country's population is now composed of 25% nonwhite individuals when considering race and ethnicity, with the nonwhite population in some states exceeding 50% [14]. Further, data indicate a decided trend in the proportion of nonwhites in the US population based on the demographics and distribution of the nation's children less than 5 years of age [27]. Such marked change in the diversity of those consuming veterinary services, directly or indirectly, is likely to bring similarly decided change in the demand or need for veterinary services. At the same time, it signals a real need to evaluate closely the diversity of the population of veterinarians to determine the likelihood of the profession's ability to continue to anticipate and meet societal needs.

A final broad-based trend specifically affecting the veterinary medical profession involves the ongoing explosion in information technology. From the increasing sophistication in computer technology available for information management on the supply side of the veterinary services market to the rapidly expanding body of knowledge accessible for consumers of veterinary services, the information age is having a profound impact on the supply and demand sides of the market for veterinarians and veterinary services. This trend enhances the quantity and quality of information available and sharply increases the speed at which information can be obtained. As such, it enhances the veterinarian's capabilities and tends to raise the bar for expected outcomes. This important trend is likely to continue into the foreseeable future.

OUTLOOK

Considering all these key trends having an impact on the market for veterinarians and veterinary medical services, the earlier contention of a complex and dynamic market seems readily apparent. With that in mind, however, certain indicators emerge relative to the outlook for the economic health of the veterinary medical profession.

First of all, the positive trend in real income for the veterinary medical profession as a whole and for new graduates is a heartening sign that signals a strengthening relation between societal needs and the services provided by the profession. Even though the debt loads of new graduates are increasing at a rate similar to the growth in these veterinarians' incomes, the growth in incomes is keeping pace. The definite positive income trend provides an encouraging outlook and stems largely from the unprecedented, and heretofore unmet, increase in demand for veterinary services. Across the spectrum, this growth in demand ranges from an increasing willingness to spend on veterinary health care on the part of animal owners to an expanding need for veterinarians in population health, public practice, research, and academia. On the clinical side, the steady growth in the demand for specialty services is particularly noteworthy, although the profession's collective ability to meet this growing demand through supplying enough specialty-trained veterinarians to meet the needs of academia and the private sector on an ongoing basis may be coming into question.

In parallel with the growth in demand, the supply side of the market also seems to be expanding. Enrollments at AAVMC member institutions are demonstrating a definite upward trend indicating increases in the number of new veterinarians entering the profession. Further, evidence indicates that veterinary practices are improving efficiency with regard to practice size and staffing patterns, thereby enabling growth in productivity for existing veterinarians. Scientific and technologic advances offer additional potential for enhancing efficiency while expanding services offered and improving outcomes.

In light of earlier claims of oversupply [1,2], this expansion on the supply side may raise some concerns. A previously published report actually challenged the validity of the claims of oversupply, however, and encouraged veterinarians to explore new opportunities through active differentiation of veterinary medical services [28]. The increasing veterinary incomes documented in the present report strongly suggest that an oversupply does not exist. Further, the increasing breadth of career opportunities available to veterinarians suggests that the issue of differentiation is, in fact, a key challenge for the future vitality of the veterinary profession. Successful innovation can, in effect, lead to creation of demand (ie, new products and services in new markets).

To meet the anticipated continued growth in demand for veterinary medical services successfully, it is crucial to meet certain ongoing challenges. As a whole, veterinarians need to continue to enhance their collective base of SKAs to appreciate and achieve fully the potential benefits offered by the unique market structure in the private practice sector and the real economic opportunities that exist across the profession. Key among these attributes should be development of the leadership skills that embody self-awareness, future thinking, team building and teamwork, communication, and the ability to develop others [21].

In addition, enhanced diversity is critical if the veterinary medical profession expects to achieve sustained success in the future. From the data presented, it is clear that the profession faces a substantial challenge related to diversity if it hopes to truly reflect the society it serves. On a positive note, the ongoing gender shift is achieving a balance between the proportion of male and female veterinarians. Trends indicate that a balance is unlikely in the longer term, however, with an ever-increasing proportion of female veterinarians. Similar imbalances exist today with regard to underrepresented minorities. Although AAVMC enrollment trends related to race and ethnicity are headed in the right direction, they are substantially behind trends in the general population. With the exception of gender, demographics of race and ethnicity are the only measures of diversity in which data exist to compare the veterinary profession with the general population; information on sexual orientation, disabilities, and other key diversity indicators are not readily available for the veterinary profession, and some measures are not even available for the general public. To understand and meet the needs of an increasingly diverse society adequately, which should help to lead to sustained success and prosperity over time, the veterinary profession must strive to be similarly diverse.

Overall, however, the economic outlook for the veterinary medical profession is strong. The market for veterinarians is not saturated; great opportunities exist, and demand is growing. Earnings in veterinary medicine may never match those possible in some other professions, but real incomes are respectable and rising across the profession, and some individual sectors can offer outstanding financial rewards. Evidence clearly indicates that the profession is increasingly valued by society, leading to the projection that economic and career prospects should continue to improve. With adequate care and forethought, veterinarians should be able to continue to meet vital societal needs in the future, and the profession should prosper and grow in the attendant rewards.

References

[1] Getz M. Veterinary medicine in economic transition. Ames (IA): Iowa State University Press; 1997. p. 13.

[2] Brown JP, Silverman JD. The current and future market for veterinarians and veterinary services in the United States. J Am Vet Med Assoc 1999;215(2):161–83.

[3] Cron WL, Slocum FV, Goodnight DB, et al. Executive summary of the Brakke management and behavior study. J Am Vet Med Assoc 2000;217(3):332–8.

[4] Volk JO, Felsted KE, Cummings RF, et al. Executive summary of the AVMA-Pfizer business practices study. J Am Vet Med Assoc 2005;226(2):212–8.

[5] American Veterinary Medical Association. Veterinary market statistics: AVMA membership (as of October 2004). 2005. Available at: http://www.avma.org/membshp/marketstats/usvets.asp#usvets. Accessed September 11, 2005.

[6] Friedman JW. Oligopoly theory. Cambridge (UK): Cambridge University Press; 1983. p. 50–75.

[7] American Animal Hospital Association. The path to high-quality care: practical tips for improving compliance. Lakewood (CO): American Animal Hospital Association; 2003.

[8] Lloyd JW, Harris DL, Marrinan MJ. Development of a veterinary teaching hospital business model. J Am Vet Med Assoc 2005;226(5):705–10.

[9] American Veterinary Medical Association. US pet ownership and demographic sourcebook. Schaumburg (IL): American Veterinary Medical Association; 2002. p. 24.

[10] Hoblet KH, Maccabe AT, Heider LE. Veterinarians in population health and public practice: meeting critical national needs. J Vet Med Educ 2003;30(3):287–94.

[11] Delgado C, Rosegrant M, Steinfeld H, et al. Livestock to 2020: the next food revolution. Washington (DC): International Food Policy Research Institute; 1999.

[12] National Research Council. Critical needs for research in veterinary science. Washington (DC): The National Academy of Sciences; 2005.

[13] Association of American Veterinary Medical Colleges. Comparative data reports, 1999–2000 through 2004–2005. Washington (DC); Association of American Veterinary Medical Colleges; 2000–2005.

[14] Association of American Veterinary Medical Colleges. DVM: DiVersity Matters. 2005. Available at: http://aavmc.org/reports_publications/documents/20050518_DVM.pdf. Accessed September 11, 2005.

[15] American Veterinary Medical Association. Veterinary market statistics: veterinary specialists. 2005. Available at: http://www.avma.org/membshp/marketstats/vetspec.asp. Accessed September 11, 2005.

[16] Lloyd JW, King LJ. What are the veterinary colleges and schools doing to improve the non-technical skills, knowledge, aptitudes, and attitudes? J Am Vet Med Assoc 2004;224(12): 1923–4.

[17] Ilgen DR, Lloyd JW, Morgeson FP, et al. Personal characteristics, knowledge of the veterinary profession, and influences on career choice among students in the veterinary school applicant pool. J Am Vet Med Assoc 2003;223(11):1587–94.

[18] Lewis RE, Klausner JS. Non-technical competencies underlying career success as a veterinarian. J Am Vet Med Assoc 2003;222(12):1690–6.

[19] Lloyd JW, Walsh DA. Template for a recommended curriculum in "Veterinary professional development and career success." J Vet Med Educ 2002;29(2):84–93.

[20] Lloyd JW, Harris DL, Marrinan MJ. Development of a veterinary teaching hospital business model. J Am Vet Med Assoc 2005;226(5):705–10.

[21] Lloyd JW, King LJ, Mase CA, Harris DL. Leadership in veterinary medicine: future needs and recommendations. J Am Vet Med Assoc 2005;226(7):1060–7.

[22] American Veterinary Medical Association. Economic report on veterinarians and veterinary practices. 2005 edition. Schaumburg (IL): American Veterinary Medical Association; 2005.

[23] American Veterinary Medical Association. Economic report on veterinarians and veterinary practices. Schaumburg (IL): American Veterinary Medical Association; 1997.

[24] Shepherd AJ. Employment, starting salaries, and educational indebtedness of year-2004 graduates of US veterinary medical colleges. J Am Vet Med Assoc 2004;224(11):1677–9.

[25] Wise JK, Adams CL. Employment, starting salaries, and educational indebtedness of 1999 graduates of US veterinary medical colleges. J Am Vet Med Assoc 1999;215(12):1783–4.

[26] Collins J. Good to great. New York: Harper Collins; 2001. p. 41–64.

[27] Hodgkinson HL. Leaving too many children behind. Washington (DC): Institute of Educational Leadership; 2003. p. 4.

[28] Lloyd JW, Smith DM. Is there an oversupply of veterinarians? J Am Vet Med Assoc 1999;216(11):1726–8.

Vet Clin Small Anim 36 (2006) 281–295

VETERINARY CLINICS
SMALL ANIMAL PRACTICE

ELSEVIER
SAUNDERS

Marketing Veterinary Services

David E. Lee, DVM, MBA

James L. Voss Veterinary Teaching Hospital, Colorado State University, 300 W. Drake Road, Fort Collins, CO 80526, USA

I n an effort to increase profitability, veterinary practice owners and managers continue to place great emphasis on financial and operational aspects—raising fees, cutting costs, and working more efficiently. Marketing, in practice, is given little consideration beyond that segment involved with promotion or advertising. Typically, discussions of marketing among veterinarians revolve around Yellow Page advertisements or cooperative arrangements with allied services. Although the promotion of services is certainly critical in generating demand for medical services, it is only one of the many aspects of marketing that ultimately determine the success of any business. Perhaps the reason why marketing as a discipline is often overlooked in the development of a business plan or practice strategy is that some elements are intuitive or perhaps incorporated in other decisions. Yet, the failure to consider marketing holistically at the onset increases the risk of implementing strategies that are disjointed and at times antagonistic.

MARKET ANALYSIS

Marketing is best considered before entering a business or adding a new service or product. Some veterinarians might have considered alternative careers had they conducted a proper market analysis before entering veterinary school. Although starting salaries for new graduates and their changes over time may be a reasonable reflection of the overall economic health of the profession, they are no more suggestive of the underlying etiology than heart rate is of cardiovascular function. Market forces shape and determine nearly every aspect of the business world in which we live and work.

Porter at Harvard University first provided an intuitive model with which to consider the attractiveness of any particular market. These forces include direct rivalry among competitors, customer bargaining power, supplier bargaining power, pressure from new entrants, and pressure from substitutes [1]. Although significant data collection and analyses may be needed to determine the impact of any of these forces on the eventual outcome of a business proposition, even

E-mail address: dlee@colostate.edu

0195-5616/06/$ – see front matter
doi:10.1016/j.cvsm.2005.11.003

casual consideration of the factors involved can greatly improve the ability to make good business decisions. Porter's Five Forces can be used to evaluate any potential market, including a new veterinary practice, service, or product. For illustrative purposes, I will use this model to evaluate the market for small animal practices as a whole but will suggest how it might be applied in other circumstances.

Direct Rivalry Among Competitors

Most practices concern themselves a great deal with the activities of their neighboring competitors. A new practice a few blocks away is likely to invoke some degree of consternation in the established practice. By definition, a market dominated by a monopoly provides little direct rivalry, whereas one shared by many companies is highly competitive. Veterinary practices continue to be small businesses, with the number of full-time equivalent veterinarians in member practices of the American Animal Hospital Association (AAHA) averaging about 2.3 [2]. Furthermore, veterinary practices tend to be rather homogenous in the types, if not the quality, of the services they provide, limited to some extent by their state's practice acts, which may dictate to some degree the services they provide and how they provide them. Consequently, veterinarians must fight for market share against a large number of rivals who may look very similar from the consumer's perspective.

Fortunately, there is greater collaboration between local veterinary practices now than in the past. Cooperation among rivals, as opposed to the constant and destructive undermining of competitors at all costs, provides the greatest possible returns to a market segment. Such cooperation is likely the result of increased emphasis on economic issues within the profession, improved business acumen among veterinarians, and enhanced communications among professionals through local and regional meetings and medical economic journals. Nevertheless, cooperation taken to its extreme is collusion, which is illegal and must be avoided. A basic and shared understanding of why fees for medical services should be high enough to recoup the significant costs of providing them is healthy for the profession, whereas an agreement made between practices regarding the fees they will charge would likely be considered collusion.

Competition for market share is less intense if the market in question is growing. The percentage of households having cats and dogs remained relatively flat in the 10 years between 1991 and 2001, yet the total number of dogs and cats increased 17% and 21%, respectively, over that time period. Total household expenditures for veterinary services increased 98% for dogs and 97% for cats [3]. On a local level, the practice owner/manager should consider local and regional demographic data in determining market size and growth. Much of this information is available free through a local chamber of commerce or via online sources. A knowledgeable consultant will be able to provide such information for a fee, although geographic information systems, discussed later in this article, may have some utility for individuals interested in applying this information on their own.

Other factors that affect direct competition include the ability of customers to "switch" between products and services. Products and services that are differentiated solely on price are called "commodities." For many consumers, the difference between leading brands of soda may be small in terms of taste. Because they usually appear side-by-side on the grocery store shelf, the "switching costs" are very low for consumers. Even more illustrative might be the situation involving milk, because most milk tastes the same to the average consumer. For that reason, most stores do not carry multiple brands of milk, and the switching cost (ie, the need to drive to a different store) is kept somewhat higher than would otherwise be expected.

Although not documented, the switching costs for clients of veterinary services have probably decreased in recent years. Improvements in medical records with the inclusion of digital images and an emphasis on documentation make it easier for one practice to assume treatment of a case seen elsewhere. Larger practices in which clients are less likely to see and bond with a particular practitioner may promote movement between practices. In general, the population seems more knowledgeable of medical issues owing to increased media attention, online information, and education, and takes a more active role in selecting and evaluating all aspects of their medical care. Continuity of care and a good relationship between the patient and physician are known to improve outcomes and decrease disenrollment in human health care [4,5].

The cost structure of a practice or a specific medical service can also affect the degree of rivalry among providers. Practices or services having high fixed costs, that is, those not affected by volume, need to maximize their use, which creates greater competition for fixed demand. A good example of this situation would be MRI capabilities in a large urban practice. The fixed costs, primarily for acquisition and maintenance agreements, are very large for MRI, and most practices offering this service require heavy use to break even. The establishment of a second unit in such an environment would initiate an aggressive struggle for market share with the likely outcome that neither practice would be able to make its financial obligations. Certainly, any means by which a practice could lower its fixed costs in such a situation, for example, through donations or grants, would impart a competitive advantage and make the decision to pursue such a service more attractive.

Competition is also impacted by a firm's ability to exit a given market with as small a penalty as possible. Given the tremendous amount of education needed, the considerable barriers to entry, and the seemingly few alternatives to clinical practice, veterinarians are unlikely to abandon practice, even in the face of low returns on investment. These factors keep competition high in an environment that would otherwise wane with greater fluidity. Barriers to exit should also be considered in evaluating new services, particularly those with high fixed costs. For example, the addition of endoscopic services should follow a reasonable assessment of the salvage or resale value of endoscopic equipment. Many practices are decorated with unused equipment purchased with the best of intentions.

Pressure from New Entrants

New entrants are attracted to a market or market segment by high returns and low barriers to entry. Finding a market that can sustain high returns while having low barriers to entry is somewhat akin to finding the "Holy Grail." A decade ago, millions of Americans were drawn to the "dot com" industry, which seemed to offer the promise of becoming a millionaire for little more investment than a home computer and a creative idea. A few creative and determined soles succeeded, but the vast majority found their ideas were quickly and easily replicated by others or more difficult to implement than they had imagined. Barriers to entry are absolutely necessary for a sustainable high return on investment.

The barriers to entry for veterinary medicine are high when one considers the amount of education required, the cost of that education, and the licensing requirements involved. Although the actual return on capital for veterinary practices has not been fully studied, some analyses assume a 12% return in determining other economic metrics, which is consistent with long-term investments in instruments carrying significantly more risk [6,7]. The return on the DVM degree has been estimated in real terms to be 9% for female and 7.7% for male graduates of colleges having average tuition costs, taking into account opportunity costs [8]; therefore, the provision of animal health services is an attractive sector.

Specialized knowledge is an effective barrier to entry, especially when regulated through licensure and accreditation. The primary intent of a state practice act is to protect the consumer and ensure that a veterinarian has the necessary level of education, yet licensing requirements and accreditation can create a barrier to veterinarians from other states or countries. If taken to the extreme, these barriers can be viewed as protectionism [9].

Probably the largest barrier to entry in an otherwise free market is imposed through economies of scale, particularly in industries having large fixed costs. Every service has a production level that maximizes efficiency, and a specific market share is required to feed that level of production. New entrants can have a difficult time achieving sufficient market share to be competitive or to meet cash flow needs in the early period. The incumbent who enjoys economies of scale also has the benefit of sharing those savings with consumers in the form of lower prices should the market become more competitive. A common mistake made by new entrants (ie, new practice owners) is to attempt to compete on price without the necessary cost structure to do so.

Pressure from Substitutes

Substitutes for veterinary services can be thought of in terms of substitutes-in-kind or substitutes-in-use. Substitutes-in-kind involve products or services that look similar and fill the same consumer need. Practice A might stock and promote antibiotic X, whereas Practice B might prefer antibiotic Y, which is virtually identical in efficacy and pharmacokinetics for use in treating the same type of infection. Substitutes-in-use fill the same consumer need but through a completely different mechanism or channel. Practice C, for example, might offer an herbal treatment that seems to be as efficacious from the client's perspective. Consumers are more likely to switch between services that are similar rather than dissimilar [10].

Substitutes for animal health care with the potential to affect a veterinary practice's market often include nonveterinarians. Animal behaviorists, chiropractors, acupuncturists, dentists, artificial inseminators, pharmacists, veterinary technicians, and farriers all have skill sets that may overlap to some degree with those of a veterinarian. Most states have practice acts that prevent these allied health providers from practicing veterinary medicine. Nevertheless, those acts are occasionally challenged, particularly as new treatment modalities not explicitly stated grow in popularity (eg, embryo transfer in cattle). Probably the most dramatic substitute for traditional veterinary care in recent years is the online pharmacy. From the client's perspective, the product they receive seems identical to that dispensed by their veterinarian, only the distribution channel has changed.

Substitutions for products and services may also occur among veterinarians. The consideration of substitutes may seem academic when evaluating the addition of a new product or service, yet some endeavors will fail if they are ignored in the process. Computers are a unique example of a technology that has simultaneously improved in quality at a high rate while decreasing in real cost to the consumer. Practices that invested large amounts of money for computer systems in the early days of computerization overcame large barriers to entry imposed by their cost. A few years later, decreasing computer costs and improved software and hardware eliminated the strategic advantages enjoyed by the early adopter.

At times, early adoption of a new technology or medical advancement can be a good strategy. The practice that pursues a particular niche, develops expertise in that area, promotes it aggressively, and, consequently, grabs the majority of market share will enjoy the barrier to entry that comes with economies of scale. The practice that adds a specialist (another form of substitute to primary care) but does not immediately leverage that advantage through promotion to and retention of referring veterinarians will quickly lose any strategic edge hoped to be gained.

Veterinarians need to be aware of potential substitutes, consider the impact to the profession and practice, and act proactively. Some substitutes have proved to be valuable allies in the provision of animal health. Licensed veterinary technicians have carved out a niche within the profession that provides improved and more efficient veterinary care. On the other hand, substitutes that find a way to circumvent barriers to entry have the ability to pluck the "low hanging fruit" from the profession.

Pressure from Buyers

The ability of consumers to dictate pricing can have a significant impact on a market. A monopoly, a market dominated by one producer, provides the consumer with little power, assuming there is a demand for the product or service and there are no substitutes. State practice acts provide a monopoly of sorts in the provision of veterinary services, which is one reason why state boards are deemed necessary to protect the consumer.

Most veterinarians have experienced the effects of buying power. Clients who constitute a large percentage of a practice's market share may have the ability to make demands for improved service or prices. A large and influential dog breeder who uses a practice's services may be more demanding than other clients. A specialist may rely on a relatively small number of practices for referrals and find they are pressured to change their operation to conform to their referring customers. If the referring practices are in a position to integrate vertically, they may change their operation to incorporate services previously required of the referral hospital (eg, hire a specialist themselves). This shift in power is especially apparent when looking at increasing competition faced by veterinary teaching hospitals.

Consumers of some veterinary services have relatively little buying power. After-hours emergencies create a situation that does not favor the client, because the switching costs (if there is an alternative) may be too high, and the clients have a critical and immediate need for emergency care.

Pressure from Suppliers

Suppliers who produce limited quantities of goods in high demand for which there are few alternatives can exert a considerable amount of power and impact a market's profitability. In the current era of "superstores" and large corporate practices, suppliers are finding themselves in the unenviable position of dealing with customers who can dictate how, when, and where they purchase their supplies. Although Wal-Mart may not be willing to pay its suppliers much in return for their goods, few manufacturers can afford to forego distribution through this channel given Wal-Mart's stranglehold on the retail market.

A large multi-practice veterinary hospital has an advantage over smaller practices because of the bargaining power they likely have with suppliers. Drug and pet food companies are more likely to sell to these practices at a discount because it is usually cheaper for them to sell in bulk as well. A very large practice can pretty much dictate the terms it has with suppliers and can play one supplier against another to extract further savings. Ultimately, smaller practices may end up paying even higher prices to offset the supplier's lost profits from larger accounts.

On a more practical scale, an investment in a new service should involve some consideration of the limits to supply. Investment in a new technology dependent on a sole source for a critical component may cause problems in the future.

MARKETING MIX

Marketers often talk about a "marketing mix" or an aggregation of attributes for a given product or service that ideally meets the needs of the client and the practice. McCarthy [11] first coined these attributes the "four P's of marketing," that is, Product, Price, Placement, Promotion. Several iterations have since been suggested for this model, including one by Lauterborn [12] that considers the marketing mix from the consumer's perspective. This latter perspective is sometimes referred to as the "four C's" of Customer solution, Cost, Convenience, and Communication. Although it is easy to see how the two models relate, there are important distinctions to be made as well.

Product

Although veterinary practices market actual physical products, the majority of their wares are medical services. The service a veterinary practice offers should be well aligned with the practice's mission, values, and strategy. Most practices strive to provide the highest quality of care, but few back up that commitment with adequate investments in continuing education, updated technology, or appropriate incentives to doctors and staff. High quality care can be expensive to provide, requiring higher fees than the practice may be willing or able to charge or collect.

As Lauterborn suggests, consumers are looking for solutions to problems. A dog scratching incessantly at its ear is a problem that needs attention. The client wants the dog to be comfortable and to stop scratching (the dog probably feels similarly). Doctor A swabs the ear, performs an excellent cytologic examination using an expensive microscope, makes the correct diagnosis, and treats the animal with the optimal antibiotic and anti-inflammatory agent. Company X may develop a new over-the-counter treatment for otitis externa that proves to be almost 100% effective, also solving the problem from the client's perspective.

The consumer approach forces the practice owner to consider what problems their clients have and to look for creative new ways to solve them. Online pharmacies are a good example. I maintain that if practice owners had been more respectful of their clients' time while they waited for medications at the end of a lengthy office visit, had done a better job of communicating the value of the medication dispensed, and perhaps not tried to subsidize the unprofitable aspects of their practices with drug sales, online pharmacies might never have gained a foothold in the market.

The KPMG LLP study surveyed pet owners to determine the top 12 factors they consider when selecting a veterinarian [13]. The top nine were ranked as follows:

> Veterinarian is kind and gentle
> Veterinarian is respectful and informative
> Reputation of veterinarian for high-quality care
> Past experience with veterinarian
> Range of services
> Location
> Convenient hours
> Recommendation from friend or neighbor
> Price

The top five considerations listed are all characteristics of the products or services that veterinarians produce. Quality is certainly one consideration but is by no means the only one or even the most important. Some practices position themselves as the "caring practice," which does get at the heart of what clients say they want most. I do not believe I have ever seen a practice that aspires to be the most "informative or respectful" clinic, and I do not think practices place enough emphasis on client retention, which is reflective of the fourth listed factor, a positive past experience.

Price

Veterinarians tend to undervalue the services they provide and, consequently, undercharge their clients. The KPMG LLP study concluded using a variety of techniques that consumers of veterinary services are relatively price insensitive, meaning that an increase in price for a given service has a comparably small impact on its demand. Fifty-eight percent of respondents agreed that they would continue to use their veterinarian even if fees were raised 20% [13].

These results suggest that veterinarians should raise fees significantly because the net response, given a consequent but modest decrease in demand, is an increased net profit, all else being equal. The ideal price for most products and services occurs at the point at which the slope of their demand curve reaches zero. Many practitioners complain of being overworked and underpaid. The logical explanation for this situation is that they simply are not charging enough. Raising fees significantly should decrease demand to a level that is more tolerable yet results in higher gross sales overall.

Although the average veterinary client may be price insensitive, such blanket statements are not true for all clients or all services. The KPMG LLP study reported that client loyalty was more pronounced for clients having household incomes exceeding $100,000 than for those making less than $40,000. As a veterinarian who has been in an examination room and discussed money with clients, I would contend that income seems to be a poor predictor of a client's willingness to purchase veterinary services. Nevertheless, for whatever reason, there is considerable variation in clients' sensitivity to fees, and this sensitivity varies with the service and situation.

Commodities are products or services that are so similar in their characteristics, regardless of their producer, that they can only be differentiated on price. As discussed earlier, milk is largely a commodity. Commodities are typically plentiful and easy to compare. Nearly all primary care animal hospitals provide surgical sterilization, and as far as the average client can tell, a spay is largely a spay. Some practices even foster the consumers' image of an ovariohysterectomy as a commodity by advertising their spay and neuter prices to help with price comparison. Although routine, an ovariohysterectomy is not minor surgery, and there can be tremendous variation in surgical preparation, technique (including laser and laparoscopic techniques), anesthetic protocols, and postoperative pain management provided by practitioners. A lack of communication of these value-added services on the part of the veterinary team fails to promote their service above the commodity status. There are very few true commodities in veterinary medicine, particularly when the product attributes most clients seek are a kind and caring environment, informative and respectful staff, and high quality service.

Not all markets are created equally either. Because commodities are also defined by being plentiful, markets oversaturated with veterinarians are apt to focus more on price. Competing on price alone is not a sustainable competitive advantage. Veterinary fees need to recoup expenses that include variable and fixed costs. Fixed costs are those that do not vary with the level of production. A practice that decides not to schedule any appointments for a given month still has a rent payment to make, salaries to pay for nonhourly staff, and maintenance agreements due for high-end equipment. Variable expenses vary with the level of production and include direct costs, such as suture material, radiographic film, diagnostic test reagents, and other supplies.

As long as a service or product recovers more than the variable cost to produce it, there is generally some basis to provide the service because it contributes toward the practice's fixed costs. The exception would be when such a service prevents the practice from offering an alternative that promises a higher gross margin. The practice that focuses solely on vaccine revenue, another potential commodity in the absence of some differentiation, is reliant on a low margin service that competes for time with higher margin services.

The point at which a given fee recoups both its variable costs and its portion of the fixed costs is referred to as the break-even point. Anything charged above the break-even point, for a given level of demand, generates profit. For price-sensitive products, the demand curve needs to be considered, because it is possible that the increased fee would decrease demand such that the product would never break even. If consumers of veterinary services are not price sensitive, this impact is reduced.

There are several ways to determine a product's price. The simplest method is termed *cost-plus pricing* and factors in the cost of producing the product but adds a set margin to cover fixed costs and profits. This method is often applied in the pricing of pharmaceuticals and other inventory in veterinary practices. It is not unusual for a practice owner/manager to simply double the wholesale cost of the product. The advantage of this method is its relative ease, assuming the true cost of the product or service is known (this is not always true with complex procedures). This method also establishes a base that protects the practice from losing money on the sale of each product. One disadvantage of this system is that there is no accounting for demand. A drug that falls out of favor over time expires on the shelf because its price was never adjusted down when demand decreased. Although selling the drug at a lower price would have sacrificed profits or even resulted in a loss, either scenario would have been preferable to discarding the entire inventory.

Many practices apply a competitive pricing model that is based on the fees charged by their competition. The success of this model depends on the sophistication of the local market and the degree of competition among competitors.

Local veterinarians who appreciate the value of the services they provide and who charge appropriately maximize the total revenue for that market. The difficulty occurs when a practice in the local market decides to compete based on price alone, perhaps because they feel they have some sustainable advantage on the cost side. Practices applying a competitive pricing model will feel compelled to follow suit, strengthening the image of veterinary services as a commodity while decreasing their net profits.

Demand-based pricing is charging what the market will bear. This method can be extremely profitable in emerging markets where clients may not have alternatives, yet it makes the market susceptible to new entrants who recognize they can offer the same service for considerably less money. Even in a price-insensitive market, clients will not tolerate price gouging for long. Practices have historically used demand-based pricing for certain services or products to help subsidize other less profitable aspects of the practice. In virtually every case, including vaccinations, pharmaceuticals, and premium diets, "cherry pickers" emerge to take advantage of these high margin markets, leaving practices to ponder their own profitability.

A more sophisticated pricing model is based on the client's perceived value of a service or product. Knowing what clients value and charging appropriately requires excellent communication, feedback by way of surveys and focus groups, and a management system sensitive enough to detect small changes in retention, market share, and product preference. If implemented, this model ensures that fees are most in tune with the market. To facilitate this process, Wutchiett Tumblin and Associates in their 2003 Companion Animal Study recommended a model that bases fees as a percentage of a practice's complete physical examination fee [14]. Although this is an impure application of value-based costing, it is a practical method of implementation.

Placement

The concept of placement is better thought of as location, convenience, or distribution for veterinary purposes. For example, a practice can provide high-quality services at appropriate prices yet be so inconvenient in terms of scheduling, accessibility, or billing that clients will seek services elsewhere. On-line pharmacies provide similar products to veterinary practices at competitive prices but do so through a convenient distribution channel—the Internet.

"Location, location, location" is a common mantra for success in business. Geographic information systems and good demographic databases can help plot competition against projected demand for veterinary services to suggest ideal locales for a new or expanding practice. A recent study showed that personal income among veterinarians was closely associated with the community size and mean household income of the practice area [15]. Nevertheless, this information should only be considered a starting point, because even the most promising location on paper can be negated by proximity to a dangerous intersection, a difficult left turn, limited parking, or other convenience factors. Practices in areas where real estate is scarce may be forced to "make do" with a building that is less than ideal in terms of location, size, and shape. Other practices become caught up in the emotion of building a practice and find themselves in the same unenviable position. Choosing a location for a practice is probably best done with the help of a knowledgeable consultant or real estate professional.

Consideration of distribution channels can lead to some interesting new niches. The veterinarian who chooses to provide high-quality medical care for cats ("product") and elects to charge premium prices can also differentiate his or her product based on distribution. A house call practice is very different from a brick and mortar practice and appeals to a very different market segment. Telemedicine, digital imaging, and the Internet are technologic advancements that have opened new distribution channels to creative practitioners.

Promotion

Although sometimes considered synonymous with marketing, promotion or advertising is only one part of the marketing mix. Promotion is important because even the ideal product at the ideal price, delivered with optimal convenience, will fail if no one knows it exists. Likewise, no degree of promotion can sell a poor product at an exorbitant price.

Practices accredited by the AAHA spend, on average, 1.1% of total income on promotion, including Yellow Page advertisements, direct mail, newsletters, and brochures. For the average size practice, this equates to a total annual expenditure of about $9500, but 25% of practices spent more than $12,000 per year [16]. Larger practices spend less on promotion as a percentage of revenue than do smaller practices, suggesting that this expense is somewhat fixed. This observation makes sense if a Yellow Page advertisement constitutes the majority of these expenditures.

Before 1977, advertising was considered an unethical practice by the American Veterinary Medical Association (AVMA) and was prohibited by most state veterinary practice acts, as well as by regulatory agencies governing attorneys and physicians. The US Supreme Court decision of Bates versus the State Bar of Arizona of that year ruled that it was unconstitutional to restrict advertising by professionals based on the right of freedom of speech [17]. Although the decision directly impacted state bar associations, the AVMA quickly concluded that the ruling also applied to veterinarians. As a result, the AVMA changed its regulations governing advertising to address ethical considerations, including false, deceptive, or misleading representations.

Although the Bates' decision makes it legal and ethical for veterinary practices to advertise, the small average annual expenditure allocated for this purpose suggests that veterinarians may feel pressured by their colleagues locally or do not expect a reasonable return on the investment. Local norms for advertising, if agreed upon, help minimize advertising expenses for the local market. The new entrant who purchases a full-page Yellow Page advertisement or advertising space in the local paper escalates total market advertising costs as others feel obliged to compete.

It is well recognized that the cost of attracting a new customer is significantly higher than the cost of retaining a current one. In one study, companies that were able to reduce customer defections by 5% realized an increase in profits between 25% and 85% [18]. This relationship is true because the cost of attracting a new client is paid upfront and amortized over the length of the relationship. Loyal clients tend to be less price sensitive and promote the practitioner's services for free. Returning customers are also easier to serve and make employees' jobs more satisfying. Overall, retaining an existing customer is about five times more profitable than attracting a new one [19].

Veterinarians have the best opportunity to promote their products and services while their client is present for a visit. A recent study by the AAHA looking at client compliance found that veterinarians failed to capture a significant amount of revenue through their failure to promote needed medical care. In the study, 50% of clients complied with the recommendations by their veterinarian for dental prophylaxis. An additional 25% would have likely complied had their veterinarian followed-up with the recommendation [20].

A logical approach for veterinarians to take in optimizing their promotional costs would be to first focus on improving client compliance for current products and services. The cost of doing so would be virtually negligible using current resources, and the potential impact on profitability could be considerable. Client compliance ensures high-quality medicine, which improves client satisfaction and loyalty. Retention measured by client visits per year rather than just the number of clients kept on the books should improve as a result. Attracting new clients through advertising is also important, but such expenditures become synergistic if compliance and retention are maximized first.

MARKET SEGMENTATION AND YIELD MANAGEMENT

The conclusions of the KPMG LLP study regarding price sensitivity tend to assume that the market for veterinary services is homogenous, which would imply that an ideal marketing mix would meet the needs of all clients. Although the consumers of companion animal veterinary medical services tend to be pet owners, the market can still be segmented into many different subgroups, each preferring its own ideal marketing mix and representing a potential niche market for veterinary services. To illustrate this principle, I will make some broad generalizations regarding segments of the veterinary market, recognizing that these representations may not hold for all markets and in all situations.

Senior citizens often depend on a fixed income for their daily needs and may not have adequate reserves to cover unexpected veterinary costs. This segment, on the other hand, may have greater flexibility in scheduling office visits during the day yet prefer not to drive during heavy traffic times or after dark. A practice wanting to focus on this market segment would do well to ensure convenient access, including provisions for disabilities. Office hours might be scheduled during the midday rather than during the morning and afternoon. The cost structure for the hospital might need to be sufficiently low to support somewhat reduced fees for this segment.

Professionals who commute from the suburbs to high-paying jobs in the city are probably less price sensitive than is the average client. Members of this segment are exquisitely time sensitive, preferring evening and weekend appointments and resenting long waits in the waiting room. The cost of extending hospital hours can be significant, yet this segment expects to pay more for this convenience, especially given the opportunity costs associated with them having to take a day off from work to seek veterinary care.

Many other segments should be considered, each with its unique needs for veterinary care. Cat owners tend to have different preferences than dog owners. Psychographic attributes can also be analyzed and targeted, with a practice perhaps positioning itself to appeal to young technologically savvy and fashion-conscious pet owners. Targeting a certain market segment and optimizing their marketing mix can give a practice an advantage over rivals who continue to be generalists.

Many practices, for business reasons alone, would prefer to serve the least price-sensitive market segments, and setting high fees can help self-select that market. The practice that finds itself with extra capacity in terms of labor or facilities may want to pursue yield management as a strategy to provide additional revenue when fixed costs are high. Yield management was implemented to great effect by the airline industry after the US Airline Deregulation Act was passed in 1978. Virtually overnight deregulation created an intensely competitive market in an industry characterized by extremely high fixed costs and considerable risk. Some airlines opted to focus solely on the business traveler who was not price sensitive (because his or her company was paying the fare) yet required more flexibility in scheduling short trips at the last minute. Other carriers continued to cater to the vacation traveler who shopped for the lowest fares but could schedule vacation flights months in advance. A third category, the budget traveler, cared little about comfort or convenience but wanted the cheapest fare possible.

The new airlines that arose from deregulation, as well as the few who survived it intact, discovered that it was possible to cater to several different market segments to fill up a plane. At some point, assuming the variable costs were met, even the addition of one discounted ticket holder contributed to the profitability of a flight. The means by which multiple market segments are pursued to optimize total revenue is termed *yield management*. A key basis for its success is the "rule of separation," which helps ensure some degree of separation between segments to discourage less price-sensitive customers from taking advantage of lower fares [21].

Airlines use differential pricing requiring a business traveler to pay a substantially higher fare than the vacation or budget traveler who may occupy the adjacent seat. It would not be practical or effective to simply ask travelers to identify themselves as a business traveler or a budget traveler before quoting a fare. Instead, the industry analyzed the needs of its passengers and realized that their consumers could be segmented into the two groups naturally by requiring a weekend night stay or 30 days' advance notice, both of which are not just undesirable for business travelers but in some cases impossible. There is little fare dilution from business travelers trying to meet the requirements for a discounted ticket; however, some budget travelers will pay higher fares when they are not able to book flights in advance.

Airlines would obviously prefer to fill their planes completely with high-paying business travelers in the same way that veterinary hospitals would prefer to fill their examination rooms with price-insensitive clients. A plane flying half full is analogous to a hospital that has empty examination rooms and idle staff at certain times of the day. If a practice can see more clients and those clients will not displace higher paying clients, yield management can help optimize revenue and ultimately profitability.

Returning to the earlier example, working professionals and senior citizens are two market segments that are easy to differentiate based on their needs and preferences. An extension of office hours into the evening and weekends would accommodate commuters. Although these services tend to be more expensive to provide owing to labor constraints, this group is presumably less price sensitive and willing to pay a premium for such convenience. Seniors may be more willing and better able to fill midday appointment slots that would otherwise go unfilled. Assuming labor and facilities are available to accommodate this demand, the practice will realize increased total revenue and profitability even if a modest discount is applied for midday appointments (making sure variable costs are covered). Each market segment obtains a product mix that is customized to them. The key is to minimize the degree to which price-insensitive clients (eg, working professionals) are displaced by price-sensitive "shoppers."

Naturally, the examples used herein are simplified and based on conjecture. In actual practice, the owners of a new hospital would need to look hard at the demographics of their area, attempt to identify discrete segments, strategize as to which segments best fit with the practice's values, mission, and resources, and conduct focus group studies to understand the needs of the proposed segments. Only then could the practice begin to apply yield management techniques to maximize profitability. Recent increases in practice revenue have largely been due to fee increases applied across the board [15]. At some point (some practices may be there already), market segmentation, price differentiation, and yield management may be necessary to further increase returns.

SUMMARY

Marketing is a holistic process that goes far beyond a Yellow Page advertisement or a glossy brochure. A thorough evaluation of a market before entry, including best and worst-case scenarios, is critical to making good investments. Veterinarians are fortunate to have a market that is largely protected by barriers to entry and characterized by reasonably high rates of return given minimal risk. Our market base continues to expand and, overall, remains fairly price insensitive. The extent to which a practice can align its capabilities with a product mix that ideally meets its clients' needs will ultimately determine its success.

References

[1] Porter ME. Competitive strategy. New York: Free Press; 1980. p. 4.

[2] American Animal Hospital Association. Staff. In: Financial & productivity pulsepoints. Lakewood (CO): AAHA Press; 2004. p. 22.

[3] American Veterinary Medical Association. US pet ownership & demographics sourcebook. Schaumburg (IL): American Veterinary Medical Association; 2002. p. 2–5.

[4] Cabana MD, Jee SH. Does continuity of care improve patient outcomes? J Fam Pract 2004;53:12.

[5] Safran DG, Montgomery JE, Chang H, et al. Switching doctors: predictors of voluntary disenrollment from a primary physician's practice. J Fam Pract 2001;50:2.

[6] Shepherd AJ. Veterinary practice expenses and financial ratios. JAVMA 2005;226:11.

[7] Wise KJ, Shepherd AJ. Revenues, expenses, and returns on resources for private veterinary practices in the United States, 2001 and 2003. JAVMA 2005;226:6.

[8] Getz M. Veterinary medicine in economic transition. Ames (IA): Iowa State Press; 1997. p. 61.

[9] Wilson JF. Law and ethics of the veterinary profession. Yardley (PA): Priority Press; 2000. p. 52.

[10] Day GS, Reibstein DJ. Wharton on dynamic competitive strategy. New York: John Wiley & Sons; 1997. p. 26–9.

[11] McCarthy EJ. Basic marketing: a managerial approach. 12th edition. Homewood (IL): Irwin; 1996.

[12] Lauterborn R. New marketing litany: 4P's passé; C words take over. Advert Age 1990;61: 26.

[13] Brown JP, Silverman JD. The current and future market for veterinarians and veterinary medical services in the United States. JAVMA 1999;215(2):166.

[14] Wutchiett Tumblin and Associates. Well managed practice study: companion animal study. Columbus (OH): Wutchiett Tumblin and Associates; 2003. p. 21.

[15] Volk JO, Felstad KE, Cummings RF, et al. Executive summary of the AVMA-Pfizer business practices study. JAVMA 2005;226(2):213, 216.

[16] American Animal Hospital Association. Expenses. In: Financial and productivity pulsepoints. 3rd edition. Lakewood (CO): AAHA Press; 2004. p. 130–1.

[17] Bates v State Bar of Arizona, No. 76–316, 433 US 350 (1977).

[18] Reichheld F, Sasser W. Zero defections: quality comes to services, Havard Business Review 1990;16:105–11.

[19] Buchanan R, Gilles C. Value managed relationship: the key to customer retention and profitability. Eur Manage J 1990;8(4):523–6.

[20] The path to high quality care: practical tips for improving compliance. Denver: AAHA; 2003. p. 80–2.

[21] Daudel S, Vialle G. Yield management, applications to air transport and other service industries. Paris: Les Presses de L'Institut du transport aerien; 1994.

Vet Clin Small Anim 36 (2006) 297–327

VETERINARY CLINICS
SMALL ANIMAL PRACTICE

Contemporary Issues of Veterinary Practice Valuation and Sale Transactions

Larry F. McCormick, DVM, MBA[a],*,
Thomas McFerson, CPA, ABV[b],
Lorraine Monheiser List, CPA, MEd[c]

[a]Simmons and Associates Mid-Atlantic, 240 Miller Lane, Boalsburg, PA 16827, USA
[b]Gatto McFerson, CPAs, 528 Arizona Avenue, Suite 201, Santa Monica, CA 90401, USA
[c]Summit Veterinary Advisors, LLC, 10354 West Chatfield Avenue, Suite 103, Littleton, CO 80127, USA

AUTHORS' COMMENTARY

From the initial invitation to author this article on practice valuation, it was our desire to use this opportunity to discuss a few significant topics that we believed were pertinent to today's veterinary practice marketplace. Of these topics, none is more important than our lead-off discussion on practices with no or little salable value. Veterinary practice appraisers are seeing a disturbing increase of seemingly healthy practices that, when appraised, are found to have little goodwill value. The circumstances underlying this problem are insidious in nature with the condition often remaining unrecognized until such time when an appraisal is performed, usually as a part of the seller's preparation for selling the practice. The discussion includes our observations on the genesis of the problem, its recognition, and corrective measures to help recover the lost practice value. This is a must read for all practice owners and buyers, especially for owners who anticipate selling their practice within the next 5 years.

The next two discussions on what is value and what influences the value of a veterinary practice and measuring a veterinary practice's value continue the initial discussion on practice value, but now the focuses are more conceptual and therapeutic in nature. Our objective is to provide the reader with a conceptual understanding of what comprises practice value, how value is created, what drives value, and, finally, how value is measured. The discussion includes a valuation worksheet designed to provide owners with a rough estimation of their practice's value; should the worksheet result be lower than expected, we

*Corresponding author. E-mail address: lmccormick@tmccg.com (L.F. McCormick).

0195-5616/06/$ – see front matter
doi:10.1016/j.cvsm.2005.10.010

encourage you to consider having a qualified professional practice appraiser develop a more complete and exact valuation of your practice.

The fourth topic of discussion focuses on the evolution of the small animal practice marketplace. This discussion examines how the marketplaces of the past have shaped our contemporary marketplace and especially addresses major changes and advancements seen in the past 15 years.

Buyers and sellers are not always sure what assets are normally included in the appraisal value and in the sale transaction. Our next discussion on assets (and sometimes liabilities) typically sold in the sale of a veterinary practice discusses the assets typically transferring in a sale transaction.

The last three topics each discuss a specific valuation issue. The discussion on the great giveaway (the costs of selling a portion of your practice) addresses the frequently overlooked and poorly understood costs associated with selling a portion of your practice to an associate. The discussion on lack of marketability discount and how this influences value deals with the issue of marketability discount and under what circumstances it is appropriate for appraisers to apply this discount. The final discussion on C corporation issues and how this may influence value is targeted for C corporation owners and addresses the unique and potentially devastating double taxation implications of selling C corporations assets.

PRACTICES HAVING LITTLE OR NO SALABLE VALUE: A DISTURBING NEW TREND

Picture yourself as a practice owner only a year away from retirement. You have spent the past 30 years of your life building a small animal practice that is now debt-free and operates from a hospital facility you own with only 5 years left on a 20-year mortgage. As the sole owner of this unincorporated business, you are taking home more than $225,000 per year from the practice. You have two associates who are interested in forming a partnership and buying your practice when you retire, and you know that your practice is valuable because of the cash you are able to pay yourself each year.

In anticipation of the sale, you hire a veterinary practice appraiser who asks you for data about your practice, analyzes that data, and gives you a report saying that your practice, which grosses $1.5 million annually, is worth only $675,000. How can that be? You say to yourself that the appraiser must have done something wrong, so you call him or her.

What the appraiser tells you is that the $225,000 you are drawing from the practice actually represents several different payments.

- First, because you are a sole proprietor and do not pay yourself a salary as an employee, part of that sum represents payment for your services as a veterinarian. Because you personally produce $375,000 annually, the appraiser tells you that 22% of $375,000 is a reasonable approximation of what it would cost to replace your production with that of an experienced veterinarian; thus, $82,500 represents payment for your services before payroll taxes.

- Second, the hospital facility was valued by a commercial real estate appraiser at $1.2 million, and fair rent on that facility was determined to be $120,000 per year. Whether you continue to own the facility and charge a fair rent to the buyers or choose to sell the real estate now, the practice has to pay rent to someone to continue to use this facility.
- Finally, the appraiser reminds you that the difference between the $225,000 you are drawing, the $82,500 for your compensation, and the $120,000 in fair rent leaves only $22,500 as the net discretionary earnings or profit from this practice, which you, as the sole owner, were entitled to take for yourself. That suggests this practice is not extremely profitable based on today's standards; a $22,500 profit on $1.5 million of gross fees represents only a 1.5% net profit, which is low for the industry. Furthermore, the appraiser reminds you that your practice's growth in gross fees, number of new clients, and average transaction charge is nominal, which you acknowledge is probably because you have been "coasting" a bit in anticipation of retirement. You have not been adjusting fees regularly as costs have risen, and you and your associates have not been as active in the community as you used to be.

Is this the kind of news you want to get just as you are ready to retire? You thought your practice was worth somewhere between $1.2 million and $1.5 million, based on gross fees. How could you have been so far off?

Unfortunately, there are a number of veterinarians who are soon going to be facing this exact scenario. Are you one of them? Later in this discussion, there is a worksheet that you can use to estimate your practice's net earnings so you know whether your earnings are closer to the $225,000 or the $22,500 in this example. In the meantime, let's explore some of the business life cycles that can occur as a practice matures.

1. Newer practice owners tend to have loans that they must repay, such as acquisition debt to buy the practice or a mortgage from buying or building a practice facility. These practices may also incur additional debt to remodel or to buy or lease new equipment in the first few years. Throughout this period, the owners are focused on profitability because they need to be sure that the practice generates enough money to service these debts.
2. As the practice matures and any acquisition or expansion debts are reduced or repaid, there are fewer demands on the practice's profits. That generally means that the owners can give themselves raises and feel less pressure to maintain or increase the bottom line. They become comfortable with the practice's financial situation as well as with their personal financial situation simply because there are fewer outsiders demanding a piece of the profits.
3. After a few years of being comfortable, the owners start coasting into retirement. They no longer read articles or attend seminars on practice management that address issues like raising fees regularly, monitoring increased costs, and reacting quickly to negative trends in profitability. Practices that are not growing can actually look more profitable on paper, simply because the equipment is older and less depreciation expense is deducted each year. That lack of growth becomes quite apparent when the practice is appraised, however.
4. The old rules of thumb about practice value do not hold true anymore. Practices do not sell based on one times the annual fees, and capitalization rates

are not always 20%. Lots of practice owners still believe that these rules govern practice valuations, however. In fact, today's veterinary practice valuations must reflect the overall economy as well as the risk associated with practices in general and with any one practice in particular.

5. Valuation theory is not static; it changes as the marketplace changes and as lenders become more or less willing to loan buyers the dollars needed to buy today's practices. Veterinary practice brokers can tell you that practices in some geographic areas are routinely worth less to buyers than practices elsewhere in the country. Some practices cannot be sold at all, except by liquidating the equipment and inventory. In fact, that is becoming an all-too-common scenario and is the worst surprise of all.

The subsequent sections of this article, especially the next two, are presented to educate you about how valuation theory has evolved, what determines value, what key factors are critical in getting top dollar for your practice, and the methods that today's appraisers use to value a veterinary practice. By understanding how an appraiser might look at your practice, you can better position yourself and your practice when the time comes to sell your practice. The steps you take now and the decisions your make in the last 3 to 5 years of practice ownership have a tremendous bearing on the value of your practice. This discussion is primarily aimed at companion animal practice owners, although some of the concepts hold true for food animal, equine, and mixed practices as well.

A successful retired former practice owner offered this sage advice: "There are two stages of practice ownership that require the owner's greatest personal investment of time and attention—the first 5 years of practice ownership as the practice is nurtured into a viable business and the last 5 years as the practice is prepared for an eventual sale." Practice owners are well advised to follow this wise veterinarian's advice.

WHAT IS VALUE, AND WHAT INFLUENCES THE VALUE OF A VETERINARY PRACTICE?

Business appraisers spend years studying and perfecting their approaches to assessing value. They take examinations, achieve credentials, and are constantly refining their craft. Appraising businesses is a never-ending journey—a field that is constantly changing and requires consistent education.

To be able to teach you, the reader, the hard calculations of appraising or to be able to give you a "how to" type of knowledge in one article would be an impossible task. The goal here, instead, is to give you an overview: to lay out the theories behind appraising a business, specifically a veterinary business. Hopefully, after reading this article, you are going to understand the concept of value as well as why one veterinary practice can have more or less value than another.

Concepts of Practice and Goodwill Value

The dictionary defines value as "the amount of money or goods or services that is to be considered the fair equivalent of something else." When a buyer purchases a practice at the stated value, what has he or she purchased? He or she has purchased the bundle of assets, including tangible assets (eg, inventory, equipment, furnishings) and, hopefully, intangible assets generally referred to as goodwill. In the successful veterinary practice, the intangible or goodwill asset is the largest asset, often accounting for 85% of the practice value.

The basis for goodwill value involves the concept of return on investment and can probably be best understood by initially looking at situations when it is not present, such as a practice that is just ready to open. The owner has made an investment in tangible assets and through effectively employing or using these assets, he or she anticipates generating an earnings stream—a return on the investment in the tangible assets. Initially, the earnings from operations are low and construed to be a reasonable return from making the investment in the tangible assets. In a successful practice, however, the earnings stream continues to grow and, at some point, the earnings begin to exceed the level of return that can be expected or explained from the investment in tangible assets. It is at this point that a new asset, an intangible asset, commonly referred to as goodwill, begins to appear. The increasing level of earnings is the outward sign of the existence or presence of increasing levels of goodwill.

From this discussion, it is important to note the following:

- Only profitable practices have goodwill.
- Goodwill is an intangible asset; as such, it is difficult to grasp the concept. It includes the practice name, reputation, location, client lists, and patient records. In the final analysis from a business value perspective, however, it is the likelihood that the clients continue to return to the practice.

Standards of Value

For appraisers, there are differing standards or rules under which value must be determined. In certain circumstances, it is possible to have two significantly differing value determinations depending on the standard of value used by the appraiser. Choosing the standard of value is one of the most critical decisions that an appraiser can make.

The two most commonly used standards of value used in valuing veterinary practices are fair market value (FMV) and investment value.

Fair Market Value

The FMV standard is defined as being the amount at which property would change hands between a hypothetic pool of willing buyers and a hypothetic pool of willing sellers when neither is acting under compulsion and both have reasonable knowledge of all the facts. In effect, the FMV standard determines value from the perspective that the practice is being marketed in a competitive environment. Generally speaking, because most veterinary appraisals are conducted for the purpose of selling 100% of the practice on the open market (ie, a competitive environment), the FMV standard is the most commonly used standard.

Investment value

The investment value standard determines value from the perspective of a specific buyer rather than a competitive pool of buyers. This standard is used to establish value in partial practice sales, such as associate buy-ins. This differs from the FMV standard in that there are no hypothetic pools of purchasers or sellers in this transaction. Rather, the buyer and seller are known, and the standard of value is to determine what the practice is worth to these specific parties. In an associate buy-in, the purchaser is buying only a piece of an existing practice and is therefore buying an undivided interest in all the assets (including cash and leasehold improvements) and taking responsibility for an undivided portion of all the practice's debts. Furthermore, the associate is not likely to be able to make significant changes as to how the practice operates (ie, increase fees, offer new services, decide to replace equipment) without the agreement of the existing owner. Similarly, the associate does not have the authority to renegotiate the lease on the practice's facility or change any of the underlying equipment leases or other financing.

What Comprises Value?

What makes something valuable? Supply and demand? Return on investment? Hard costs already spent? Compensation for time and sweat equity? All these items play a role in determining the value of something.

Of course, what ultimately determines the value of a veterinary practice is what someone is willing to pay for it. Why can two practices with similar tangible assets have differing value determinations? Many factors interrelate to determine what a buyer is willing to pay for a practice. For appraisal purposes, these factors can be distilled down to two predominant factors that drive the value of a practice: the ability of a practice to generate an expected level of earnings or cash flow (called the benefit stream) and the risks associated with the practice's ability to continue to generate that expected benefit stream consistently in the future. Let's look at these two factors in greater detail.

Expected cash flow

Expected cash flow can be defined as revenues less all the customary operating expenses, including fair compensation for the owner and/or doctor. Restated, it is the discretionary cash flow expected to be available to owners as a result of operating this practice.[a] Generally speaking, a veterinary practice with a higher cash flow has a higher value. A practice with a lower cash flow understandably has a lower value. Because veterinary practices have little in the way of hard assets (eg, inventory, equipment), the cash flow is the overwhelming majority of what a buyer is buying.

Risk

The second major component of value is the financial risk involved in owning and operating a veterinary practice. More specifically, from an appraisal perspective, it is the risk associated with the ability to deliver the expected cash flow or benefit stream. Appraising the risks involved is one of the arts that

---

[a] The terms *expected cash flow, discretionary cash flow, benefit stream, expected earnings,* and *return on investment* all refer to the same number or value. Although they are interchangeable, each does provide a slightly varying perspective.

an appraiser must master. Looking at a practice and determining where the risks lie is an important part of the process. Many appraisers have a checklist of different aspects of veterinary practices that they grade and analyze. The better these are, the lower the risks involved. The lower the risks involved, the more a buyer would be willing to pay.

MEASURING VETERINARY PRACTICE VALUE IN TODAY'S MARKETPLACE

As was suggested in the opening pages of this article, many practices today have little salable value. Although these practices may have provided the owner with a reasonably good job and a moderately comfortable lifestyle, these practices are not able to generate a reasonable return on investment or adequate levels of earnings or profits. The terms *return on investment, earnings,* and *profits* all mean exactly the same thing—the money remaining after paying the operating expenses of the practice and after paying the owners for their efforts as veterinarians and managers. For a practice to have salable value, it must generate a sufficient amount of earnings (or profits or return on investment). The greater the level of earnings or profits, the greater is the return on investment and the greater is the salable value of the practice.

Today's purchasers are looking at return on investment, that is, they are relating the income they can expect to receive from a practice to the cost of buying it. If that relation does not make sense, they are going to look for another practice to buy. For the deal to work, the buyer must be able to use the practice's income from fees and services to pay all the normal operating expenses, pay the buyer for his or her veterinary production and management efforts in the practice, cover the payments that are owed to the lender who advanced the funds to buy the business, and still have enough dollars to reinvest in new equipment and practice growth.

That means that buyers and sellers need to understand some basic valuation concepts, such as capitalization and discount rates, benefit streams, the difference between profit and cash flow, and how risk affects value.

First, however, there are a few general valuation concepts that you need to understand. There are three basic valuation approaches that a business appraiser can use to measure a practice's value: the market approach, the asset approach, and the income approach:

1. The market approach suggests that a business might be valued by pricing it like comparable businesses that actually sold on the open market. There are at least two major obstacles related to veterinary practices, however. Conceptually, are any two veterinary practices really comparable? This approach assumes that there is more similarity between businesses in the same industry than we generally find in veterinary practices. The greater problem has been that almost all veterinary practice sale transactions are between private parties. Consequently, there have been no reliable data available to appraisers to analyze actual transactions in the marketplace. Such a database is in the early stages of development by the Association of

Veterinary Practice Management Consultants and Advisors and may some-day make this approach possible; however, for now, veterinary appraisers are unable to use the market approach effectively.

2. The second approach, the asset approach, determines value by summing the current value of each and every asset and liability that belongs to the busi-ness. If veterinary practices were like a holding company that consisted solely of publicly traded stocks, we could determine the current price of each security that the business owns. Then, by adding up all the current val-ues and subtracting any outstanding debts, we would have the value of the total portfolio and of the business. Veterinary practices are quite different, however. Although each practice owns equipment, inventory, furniture, and supplies, for example, that could theoretically be valued, most of the true worth is in the intangibles (ie, goodwill, going concern value) that are represented by the profits, client list, patient records, and other assets, which are difficult to value. Therefore, the asset approach is generally only used when a veterinary practice is being liquidated (ie, shut down) because the owner has left the practice without finding a buyer and the only remaining value is in the inventory and equipment, which might be useful to another practice.

3. The third approach, the income approach, determines value based on a busi-ness's ability to generate income—generally, bottom line profits with certain modifications. This approach bases value on the historical benefit stream or, alternatively, on the anticipated benefits that a business is expected to generate.

In valuing veterinary practices, the income approach is most commonly used together with a method involving the capitalization of an income or benefit stream to determine all or part of the value of the practice. One or both of these two methods are generally used to value veterinary practices. These capitaliza-tion-based methods are the single period capitalization (SPC) method and the excess earnings (EE) method.

If a single capitalization rate is applied to the entire benefit stream, the ap-praiser is using the SPC method. This presumes that the benefit stream results from use of the entire pool of assets, and it does not matter whether those assets are tangible (eg, equipment, inventory) or intangible (eg, goodwill, going con-cern value). The point is that whatever the mix of assets, they are generating the benefit stream, and thus the value of the practice.

Another variation of the income approach is the EE method. In this case, the benefit stream is divided into two pieces under the theory that part rep-resents a return on investment for the tangible assets (eg, equipment, inven-tory) and part relates to the intangibles (eg, goodwill, going concern value). The appraiser subtracts a reasonable return on the tangibles (perhaps 10%–12% annually) from the total benefit stream and then divides the remaining benefit stream by a capitalization rate that reflects the higher risk associated with intangibles. That result represents the value of the intangibles, which is then added to the value of the tangible assets in determining the total value of the practice.

Fig. 1 provides an example of how the two methods might work for the same practice. There are several important concepts inherent in these examples.

- If correctly applied, either method produces an appropriate valuation conclusion. Both methods are based on the earnings (benefit stream) that flow to the owner(s) of the practice.
- In special circumstances, the discounted future earnings method may be more appropriate than either of the capitalized earnings methods. An example might be a practice that has only a couple of years of history and has been growing rapidly. In such a case, projecting future earnings might be more appropriate than trying to determine a reasonable historical benefit stream.
- The appropriate capitalization rate varies from practice to practice because it is a reflection of risk, which is not the same in all practices. For example, a stable practice with an established clientele in a growing area inherently has less risk (and a higher value) than a practice that has experienced lots of staff turnover and is located in an area with one major employer that was just acquired by a competitor in another state.
- There is a difference between net income (or profit) and the benefit stream discussed previously. Generally, adjustments have to be made to reported net profit to adjust for reasonable owner(s)' compensation, fair rent, nonrecurring income or expense, and discretionary spending, for example. There is more information elsewhere in this article about these adjustments.
- Because the benefit stream is divided into two pieces, only one of which is capitalized in determining the value of the goodwill under the EE method, the EE capitalization rate is always different from the one used in the SPC method. Furthermore, the SPC rate is generally lower than the EE capitalization rate.
- A lower capitalization rate results in a higher figure when a benefit stream is capitalized. For example, a 20% capitalization rate translates to a multiple of 5 (1 divided by 0.20). A 25% capitalization rate is equivalent to a multiple of 4 (1 divided by 0.25).

Excess Earnings Method		
Earnings (Benefit Stream)		181,400
Value of tangible assets	145,000	
(X) Rate of return from investing in the		
tangible assets	12.0%	
Return from tangible assets	17,400	
(-) Amount of benefit stream		
attributable to the tangible assets	17,400	(17,400)
Amount of benefit stream		
attributable to the intangible assets		164,000
(÷) By the Capitalization rate for INTANGIBLE assets		22.3%
Value of intangible assets (Goodwill)		735,426
(+) Add back the value of the tangibles		145,000
Total value of all assets		880,426
Total Value (rounded)		880,000

Single Period Capitalization Method	
Earnings (Benefit Stream)	181,400
(÷) Capitalization rate for ALL Assets	20.6%
Total value of all assets	880,583
Total Value (rounded)	880,000

Fig. 1. Comparison of methods.

Calculating the Appropriate Benefit Stream (adjusted earnings)

All the valuation methods described here rely on calculating an appropriate benefit stream, which is then discounted or capitalized as appropriate. Although a complete analysis of how and when to adjust reported earnings is beyond the scope of this discussion, certain areas are especially critical and can have a major impact on a practice's value.

1. Depreciation expense: one of the adjustments that appraisers routinely make is to adjust net income to something closer to cash flow, which includes adding back any expenses that did not require cash. When a practice acquires equipment, the cost of that equipment creates an asset that is reflected on the balance sheet rather than on the profit and loss statement. That cost is then written off over the useful life of the equipment, with a portion deducted each year as an expense called depreciation. No check was written for that depreciation expense, however, and any cash that changed hands was in the year of acquisition. Therefore, depreciation expense is routinely added back to net income in calculating the benefit stream. Appraisers then subtract an amount that better represents the actual consumption and replacement of furniture and equipment.

2. Owner(s)' compensation: many factors affect how and the amount that owners pay themselves. For example, sole proprietors like the owner in our first example do not pay themselves a salary. Rather, they are taxed on all the practice's net profits for the year, and they pay themselves periodically by writing a check (with no tax withholding) to themselves. Contrast that to the owners of a C, or regular, corporation, who regularly pay themselves salaries equal to 100% of the corporate net profits for the year to avoid corporate taxation at the maximum corporate rate. For the sole proprietor, owner's compensation on the profit and loss statement is zero, whereas it is likely a large number on the C corporation's tax return. An appraiser must adjust one or both of these to represent the fact that owners are entitled to be paid for their veterinary production and for their services as the practice leader. After all, if the owner left the practice, someone with comparable skill and experience would have to be paid a fair salary to do this work.

3. Rent: if a practice rents its hospital facility from an unrelated third party, we can probably assume that the rent is close to market rent, because neither the landlord nor the practice would likely give the other party a sweetheart deal for any significant period. Conversely, if the practice owner(s) also own the real estate, the rent being paid might be anywhere from significantly less than reasonable to thousands of dollars over market rent. Therefore, an appraiser looks closely at the actual rent being paid and then determines whether that figure should be adjusted up or down to calculate an appropriate benefit stream to be capitalized.

4. Discretionary spending: owners can certainly choose what to do with the profits from their practices, but that does not necessarily mean that a buyer would make the same decisions. For example, if the seller puts his college-aged children on the payroll to provide them with spending money and an individual retirement account contribution each year, the appraiser would look closely at this arrangement. If the children are providing actual services and being paid a reasonable sum for doing so, the appraiser might make no

adjustment. More frequently, however, the appraiser would add back all or a portion of these wages as discretionary spending by the owner and as an expense that would not continue once the buyer took over ownership.

5. Nonrecurring income and expense: alternatively, a practice sometimes has income from an unusual source or an extraordinary expense that must be removed in determining the benefit stream. For example, suppose a practice has a fire that does extensive damage. The loss is covered by insurance, so the practice has the repairs made in the last few months of the taxable year. Early in the following year, the insurance company settles and sends a large check to the practice. In the first year, part of the repairs and maintenance expense would have to be removed from the benefit stream because they are nonrecurring (hopefully). In the second year, the insurance reimbursement would also be removed, because that is not normal practice income a buyer could expect to receive each year.

6. Interest or dividend income and interest expense: some practices keep their cash cushion in interest-bearing bank accounts or in taxable money market funds. The income generated from those investments relates to the owner(s)' decision to keep those funds in the practice but cannot be expected to be available to a purchaser of the practice unless he or she also has extra cash on hand (not likely in the early years). Similarly, some owners avoid practice debt and choose to fund the practice with their own money rather than incurring interest charges on borrowed funds. Others prefer to use "other people's money" and are willing to take on substantial practice debt. Therefore, interest expense for the buyer is a function of how the buyer funds the practice and is different from how the practice has operated in the past. An appraiser takes out interest or dividend income and adds back interest expense in determining the benefit stream for valuation purposes.

Although these items are not a complete list of the adjustments that an appraiser might make, they represent the most common ones. Armed with this background, you can use the following worksheet (Fig. 2) to make a quick estimate of what the benefit stream and value of your practice might be currently. If you do not like the result, now is the time to do something about it rather than when you are ready to retire.

EVOLUTION OF THE SMALL ANIMAL PRACTICE MARKETPLACE

Sellers and buyers of small animal veterinary practices are naturally concerned with how practice values are determined and the available means to finance the sale transaction. The small animal practice marketplace has evolved over several decades, with the most significant changes occurring in the past 15 years. Today's marketplace is far more sophisticated than the methods and markets of the past. Yet, the past still influences perceptions today. Looking at the past helps us to understand better what is happening now and what may happen tomorrow.

Birth of a New Industry

The advent and growth of veterinary practices dedicated exclusively to the medical and surgical care of small or companion animals have been remarkable. In the space of a few decades, small animal exclusive practices went

Worksheet to Estimate the Annual Benefit Stream (Earnings)	
Net income per books (from the tax return or profit and loss statement)	xxx
Add back non-cash expenses	
+ Depreciation expense	xxx
+ Section 179 expense (first year writeoff)	xxx
+ Amortization expense	xxx
Less economic wear & tear on equipment and furniture	
- 10% of the current value of equipment and furniture	(xxx)
Adjust owner(s)' compensation	
+ Actual owner(s)' compensation	xxx
+ Estimated payroll taxes on actual owner(s)' compensation (8%)	xxx
- 22% of owner(s)' actual veterinary production	(xxx)
- Estimated payroll taxes on estimated owner(s)' compensation (8%)	(xxx)
Adjust for reasonable rent on the practice facility	
+ Actual rent paid	xxx
- Reasonable annual rent (10% of current value of real estate)	(xxx)
Adjust for owner(s)' discretionary spending	
+ Owner(s)' non-business expenses	(xxx)
Adjust for non-recurring income and expense	
- Non recurring income	(xxx)
+ Non recurring expense	xxx
Adjust for interest/dividend income and expense	
- Interest and dividend income included in practice net income	(xxx)
+ Interest expense	xxx
Equals = Estimated benefit stream	xxx

Rough Estimate of Practice Value	
Estimated benefit stream (see above)	xxx
÷ 21% capitalization rate (assumed)	21%
= Rough estimate of practice value	XXXXXX

Fig. 2. Worksheet to estimate the annual benefit stream.

from virtual nonexistence to being the major component of the veterinary industry. Pioneer small animal practices began appearing in the 1930s and 1940s, primarily in the coastal states. This beginning was followed by a period of dramatic expansion in the number of small animal practices during the 1950s and 1960s. Many factors interacted to encourage this migration from the more traditional large animal or mixed animal practice to the exclusive small animal practice, including improved working conditions, decreased work hours spent in practice, the ability to practice a higher level of veterinary medicine, opportunity to specialize in one area of medicine or in services to one species, and improved financial success.

It is not surprising that the same attributes that encouraged veterinarians to make the transition to small animal exclusive practice also attracted potential buyers to purchase established small animal practices, fostering a competitive marketplace for owners and buyers. Within that earlier marketplace, as in today's, there were two main issues in every transaction: how the practice's transaction value was determined and how the transaction was to be financed. The evolution of these two components of every sale transaction—transaction price and transaction financing—is the focus of the balance of this discussion.

Evolution of Determining the Transaction Price

The manner of determining a practice's value for sale transaction purposes in the past was markedly different from the methods for determining value in today's marketplace. For these pioneer practices, there were no guidelines and there was no historical transaction information available to assist sellers and buyers in establishing a fair price. Most likely, these early practice transactions were based on the value of the tangible assets (eg, inventory, equipment, furniture) plus an amount to acknowledge the business as a going concern (goodwill)—in essence, a guessed price on which both sides agreed to transact.

Rule-of-Thumb Era

Gradually, and over time, various rules of thumb evolved, although just how is not clear. Nevertheless, various rules were developed over time, and they formed the basis for many small animal practice sale transactions. Most of these rules of thumb were easily understood formulas that defined practice value as a multiple of revenue. An excellent example is the most quoted of these rules of thumb: "The price of a practice is equal to the most recent year's revenue."

The relatively simplistic nature of these rules is somewhat deceptive. When the various rules of thumb are reviewed, it seems that the rules deal only with the transaction price, with no outward reference as to how the transaction is to be financed. From discussions with veterinarians who have sold their practice under one of these rules, however, it seems that there were two additional generally unstated conditions that were integral to the success of the rules of thumb.

Condition 1: loan payment period must be extended
An essential component of almost all transactions conducted under the revenue-based rules of thumb was an extended loan payment period, generally for 7 to 10 years and sometimes longer. The long loan payment periods ensured that the monthly loan payment was low enough to allow the buyer to have enough money to make payments from normal practice operations. The importance of the extended loan payment period is discussed later in this article.

Condition 2: seller financing was normally required
Because local community-type banks typically required 75% or more of the face amount on a commercial loan to be secured by collateral tangible assets (eg, equipment, inventory), they played almost no role in financing veterinary practice transactions. Typical of most service-based businesses, successful small animal practices have tangible asset bases of approximately 10% to 20% of the

total, with the bulk of the value being the intangible assets, such as goodwill. Because of this, most buyers were unable to secure commercial financing. Consequently, in almost all sale transactions, the seller simply assumed that he or she would have to provide the necessary financing to make the transaction happen. As the primary lender, the seller was able to provide the necessary longer loan payment period discussed in condition 1.

These two conditions were essential for the buyer to have sufficient cash flow to transact using the rule of thumb value determination. More importantly, as is discussed later in this article, these two conditions continue play a significant role in stabilizing value within of the contemporary practice marketplace.

Shortcomings of the Rules of Thumb

Even though these rules were used extensively for establishing small animal practice value, they did not always result in an equitable or fair transaction value. Two of the more significant problems associated with rules based on revenue production include the following:

- Rules of thumb that were based on a practice's revenue-producing capabilities assumed that all practices generating similar levels of revenue are homogeneous. In other words, practices generating the same revenue would be equally desirable to a buyer. In reality, however, buyers would always choose one practice over another for other reasons even if their gross revenue were the same. Practices are far from being homogeneous.
- Most rules of thumb were based on a multiple of gross revenue and gave no consideration to the earning-generating capabilities of a practice. The revenue-based rule implies that all practices generating the same level of revenue would produce similar levels of earnings or profits. This, of course, is far from the truth. Modern valuation methods used to value veterinary practices focus on earning generation rather than revenue. These newer methods are discussed in the next section.

Despite these major shortcomings, the 1-year's revenue rule of thumb and other similar rules remained the mainstay approach used to establish practice value until the 1980s, when business valuation methodologies began to be applied to small animal practice transactions.

Modern Business Valuation Theory

As early as 1977, there were efforts to develop a valuation approach that was grounded in the same valuation theory as was used outside the veterinary profession for other small and professional service businesses. In 1987, *Veterinary Economics* published a series of three articles describing the application of an income-based business valuation method as a viable approach to value small animal veterinary practices [1–3]. This method was the EE method. The EE method was not new; in fact, the method had been used for other kinds of small business appraisals since the days of prohibition. The *Veterinary Economics* EE method articles were one of earliest applications of a more sophisticated valuation method based on established valuation theory for veterinary practices, however. After their publication, the EE method gained favor among veterinary practice consultants and business appraisers and soon displaced the rules of thumb to become the primary method for appraising veterinary practices.

The acceptance of the EE method was driven by the fact that a more equitable practice value was likely to result by downplaying the gross revenue and focusing instead on better predictors of the future financial health and profitability of the practice. Under the EE method, practice value was determined by assessment of two key value determinants: the earnings-generating capacity of the practice adjusted by the appraiser to reflect economic reality and the risk associated with the practice's ability to produce or deliver this level of expected earnings. The EE method's ability to assess earnings and risk was a major advancement over the revenue-based rules of thumb.

In the mid-1990s, a second earnings-based method, the SPC method, began to be applied to value small animal practices. The SPC methodology is similar to the EE method because both rely on the assessment of earnings-generating capabilities and an assessment of the risk associated with producing that level of earnings. In fact, because each method develops an opinion of value from somewhat differing perspectives, it is not unusual today for appraisers to use the EE and SPC methods in the same appraisal assignment.[b]

The likelihood of accurately determining a fair and equitable transaction price for small animal practices has dramatically improved since the early days of the profession. For more than 10 years, practice appraisers and consultants have lectured on the inaccuracies of the old revenue-based rules of thumb and, in particular, have emphasized that the "1 year's gross" rule tends to overvalue today's practice significantly. At a recent American Veterinary Medical Association (AVMA) lecture, the lecturer asked an audience of approximately 60 primarily practice owners for a show of hands if they were aware of the old 1 year's gross revenue rule of thumb. Everyone attending was aware of the rule. Next, the lecturer asked how many believed this rule applied to their practice and that their practice would sell for 1 year's gross revenue. Approximately 25 people raised their hand. It seems that the old rule of thumb continues to taint the thinking and expectations of many veterinarians. This old rule seems to have a life of its own.

Evolution of the Financing Alternatives

Era of owner financing

As discussed previously, the seller traditionally provided the financing for virtually all practice sale transactions. Indeed, with few exceptions, sellers assumed the role of the primary lender for approximately the first 70 years

---

[b]The EE and SPC methods are explained in more detail in the previous discussion on measuring veterinary practice value in today's marketplace.

of the profession. It was not until the mid-1990s that alternative sources of financing began to appear.

Era of third-party financing

Practice consolidators. One of the first alternatives to traditional seller financing was with the advent of the practice consolidators (ie, national or regional entities that planned to own and operate a number of practices rather than just one or two). These consolidators first started to purchase practices in the late 1980s, but it was not until the 1990s that the consolidators began to acquire significant numbers of practices.

Some consolidators had cash available to purchase practices outright, whereas others offered various financing packages to sellers that might include cash, promissory notes, an equity interest in the consolidator, and other creative financing ideas. Although some were more successful than others, collectively, the consolidators were the first to provide selected sellers another option in addition to seller financing for exiting their practices.

Cash flow lender. In the mid-1990s, the US economy and the US stock market were functioning at all-time highs. This created the unusual situation in which many businesses, especially investment and banking institutions, had more dollars than they had safe places to invest them. They needed relatively safe investments in which to park some of these excess dollars. A few financial institutions began exploring innovative lending programs to various health professionals, in particular, funding the purchase of established practices. For the most part, these lenders ignored collateral assets as the basis for their debt exposure, focusing instead on the practice's ability to generate earnings or cash flow. As a group, these cash flow lenders found this new market profitable and safe. This was especially true for dental and veterinary practice purchase transactions, where the lenders experienced only occasional loan defaults.

As a means of lowering their risk exposure or to fund transactions that otherwise might be considered too risky, some lenders would structure financial packages to meet the necessary criteria to be guaranteed by the Small Business Administration (SBA). Over time, the SBA has modified its rules and increased the maximum amount of the loan that can be guaranteed. As a result, these loans have become ever more popular, in spite of the high loan fees built into their loan offerings.

For the seller, the advent of corporate consolidators and especially the cash flow lenders into the veterinary practice marketplace effected a remarkable 180° reversal from their historic responsibilities. No longer was the seller obligated to be the primary risk taker and provider of the long-term debt necessary to underwrite the sale transaction for a practice. Instead, with the cash flow lender now funding the sale transaction with outside debt capital, for the first time, today's seller can expect to receive most, and sometimes all, of the proceeds from the sale of his or her practice at the time of closing.

Importance of the Extended Year Loan Payment Term

The importance of an extended loan payment term in past, present, and probably future veterinary practice marketplaces cannot be overstated. When and under what circumstances the extended repayment period was first incorporated as a part of the seller's lending package for the buyer is not known, but there is little doubt that this long-term financing has been an integral component of rules of thumb–based practice transactions for several decades. Even in recent years, as the cash flow lender has quietly replaced the seller as the primary lender in a veterinary sale transaction, this extended loan term has virtually continued unchanged. Most readers of this article likely do not perceive the 7- to 10-year repayment period to be exceptionally long. It was and is just the normal way the debt associated with practice sales is structured. In comparison, however, outside of the veterinary marketplace, most small service-oriented businesses transact the sale of their businesses over a much shorter time frame, typically 3 to 5 years. Why is this difference important?

The issue is basically cash flow. When structuring a loan package, there are three major variables that can be altered to vary the monthly payment and thereby affect business cash flow: the loan principal amount, the interest rate, and the repayment term. In general, small variations made in the interest rate produce only a relatively minor change in the monthly payment. By contrast, manipulation of the loan principal amount or the repayment term has a significant impact on the monthly payment. In past eras, when using rules of thumb to establish transaction value, buyers and sellers realized early on that most practices could support a price based on the most used rule (price equals 1 year's revenue) only if a significantly longer loan repayment period was included in the loan terms. By extending the repayment term to approximately 10 years, the sellers (lenders) offered a low enough monthly payment that almost all practices would be able to cash flow the buy-in.

Was the implementation of the extended repayment period simply a process that has provided an artificial way to justify and maintain high-end value determinations of veterinary practices for decades? Although potentially true, it seems unlikely that the veterinary practice markets (buyers and lenders) would be continuously fooled over the many decades that the extended repayment period has been in place. Further, it also seems even more unlikely that the earnings-based methods of establishing business value in common use today would not have uncovered the artificial value determinations.

There is an alternative to consider that may more properly explain this situation. Consider that perhaps the 5-year or less repayment term, which is constantly referred to as being the norm, may be inappropriately short for the low-tangible asset high-goodwill service businesses like small animal veterinary practices. Perhaps, to capture the highly intangible goodwill value adequately, a longer repayment window is not only necessary but is a more appropriate repayment period. There is evidence to support this rationale: in the sale of medical practices, only two types of medical practices, the dental practice and the small animal veterinary practice, have been able to sell significant levels of intangible or goodwill value in their routine practice sale transactions successfully. For both of these professional practice types, the transaction price is largely made up of intangible assets and the lending package routinely transacts over the extended repayment time frame of 7 to 10 years.

Although generally underappreciated, the loan repayment term plays a major role in the pricing and stability of the veterinary transaction marketplace. It is absolutely essential that the extended repayment period of 7 to 10 years continue as an integral component of veterinary practice sale financing to keep practice values at the current levels.

Today's Dynamic Practice Marketplace: Evolution Continues

The veterinary practice market continues its evolution. We currently are experiencing major changes that are likely to have an impact on the marketplace long into the future.

Third-party or cash flow lenders

Without question, the advent and subsequent apparent success of lenders that base lending decisions on cash flow–generating capabilities rather than collateral have influenced the veterinary practice marketplace more than any other event. Their apparent success suggests that they are likely to continue to make loans within the veterinary practice marketplace, although they have an increasing ability to control payment terms and, indirectly, practice values. Their presence as the primary lenders at the moment affects the veterinary practice marketplace in several ways:

- Sellers are now relieved of their historical responsibility of underwriting the long-term financing of the sale. In most cases, they are now able to receive most, and sometimes all, of the sale proceeds at the time the transaction closes.
- For the first time, the presence and resources of the commercial banking industry are brought into the veterinary sale marketplace.
- These lenders have a normalizing effect on the marketplace and provide stability as long as the conditions and loan requirements remain static.

Business appraisal

The science of business appraisal continues to evolve. The sophistication of the veterinary practice appraisal environment is dramatically reaching higher levels of competence as an increasing number of individuals are pursuing courses of study toward attaining specialized credentials in the appraisal science. This sophistication of appraisers also tends to have a stabilizing effect on the marketplace.

Opportunities for younger graduates

Because of the availability of financial and business management programs as part of their veterinary school coursework, future graduate veterinarians should be more prepared for the business side of veterinary medicine and for eventual practice ownership than past generations of graduates. These veterinarians should be better managers and operators of the business side of the practice and are likely to pursue practice ownership as a business and strive to obtain a reasonable return on their investment rather than as a means of buying themselves a job.

Corporate consolidators

The corporate consolidators continue to operate with varying degrees of success in implementing their respective consolidation models. Their role in the practice marketplace is varied. Some of the consolidators have stopped or severely restricted acquisition of additional practices. Those consolidators still acquiring practices are doing so with increased selectivity. Currently, the consolidators continue to represent an alternative buyer for sellers who own practices that meet the consolidators' criteria.

Importance of maintaining practice profitability

As discussed at the beginning of this article on contemporary issues in practice valuation, practice appraisers are seeing an increased incidence of practices that seem healthy and viable on the surface but have poor or no salable value when appraised. At the heart of this problem is the failure of practice owners and managers to maintain the profitability of their practices, especially as they approach their latter years of practice. Making owners aware of the presence of this deceptively covert poor profit and poor practice value circumstance was one of the prime reasons for writing this article.

The issue of maintaining profitability is a continuous objective throughout the life of a practice. Profit is not only important for maintaining practice value but is, of course, a major key to maintaining all levels of practice vitality. Owners and managers of veterinary practices owe it to their clients to charge them high enough fees for their services so that adequate profits are made. It is these profits that enable reinvestment back into the practice to improve technology and maintain high levels of patient care. When the time comes to market the practice, these same profits ensure that it sells at a reasonable value for the seller and allow the buyer to pay off the acquisition debt. The day may come when profit is not considered a dirty word.

For 5 to 6 decades, little change occurred in the veterinary practice sale transitions in which price was primarily based on revenue-based rules of thumb and buyer's financing was almost always provided by the seller. In the past 15 to 20 years, the pace of change increased significantly, with the marketplace experiencing significant and important advancements manifested by modern business valuation methods replacing the rules of thumb as the primary means of determining practice value and commercial cash flow lenders replacing the sellers as the primary finance provider. The marketplace continues to evolve. History may well record this modern era as the era of maturation and sophistication of the veterinary practice marketplace.

ASSETS (AND SOMETIMES LIABILITIES) TYPICALLY SOLD IN A VETERINARY PRACTICE SALE

In today's market, more than 90% of all veterinary practice transactions (where the entire ownership of the practice actually changes hands) are asset sales. Few practice owners are able to sell the stock in their corporations. Even so, whether structured as a stock sale or an asset sale, the assets expected to change hands when a veterinary practice is sold remain the same—all operational assets and all clients are usually assumed to be part of the transaction.

So what are those assets that are typically included in a sale transaction or in an appraiser's value determination? What is the prospective buyer actually buying?

A veterinary practice has tangible assets and intangible assets. Tangible assets are the physical assets of a practice that can be seen or touched, such as inventory, medical equipment, or office fixtures. Intangible assets can be defined as the assets of a company that are nonphysical in form yet hold value and are crucial to the company. An example of an intangible asset would be goodwill.

Because a veterinary practice is a service business as opposed to, say, manufacturing, most of the value is placed on the intangible assets. Most veterinary practices have a moderate amount of equipment, a moderate amount of inventory, and a moderate amount of accounts receivable. But those are not generally the most important assets from a buyer's perspective. What veterinary practices do have, usually in abundance, are clients with pets, the patients of the practice. Those clients, the patient records, and the practice's reputation are valued collectively as goodwill, an intangible asset.

When a buyer buys a veterinary practice, he or she expects to buy the client-patient database and all the tangible assets needed to run the practice and service those clients adequately. What assets are those? Using the typical balance sheet of a veterinary practice as our guide, let's find out.

Current Assets

Cash or cash equivalents

Any cash on hand on the date of sale belongs to the seller. For a veterinary practice sale, cash is almost always not calculated into the overall value of the practice, and is therefore not transferred to the buyer. An exception would be a partial buy-in by an associate. In this circumstance, cash and cash equivalents less than the current liabilities remain with the practice entity; only cash and cash equivalents in excess of current liabilities stay with the seller.

Accounts receivable

The accounts receivable asset is usually handled differently than the other assets of a practice. The receivables are usually not included in the value determination made as a result of the normal appraisal process. The asset is frequently included in many sale transactions as a discounted add-on, however. The amounts shown in the accounts receivable represent as yet unpaid revenues previously generated for services performed by the seller. To make the transition easier for the buyer and seller, the accounts receivable asset is discounted to an amount estimated to be actually collectible. This discounted amount is subsequently added to the transaction and transferred to the buyer as part of the sale transaction. The buyer then is entitled to keep whatever is ultimately collected.

Inventory

The inventory usually comprises the medical supplies, pet food, over-the-counter products, surgical supplies, and other items used in the day-to-day treatment of animals. This asset is absolutely transferred to the buyer. Usually, it is up to the buyer and seller to agree on the overall cost of the inventory to be transferred on the day of sale. A count is done by the buyer and seller 48 hours before the sale to determine how much actual inventory is on the shelves. If the inventory cost is within 10% of the agreed-on value, no adjustment is needed. If there is more of a disparity, an adjustment to the sales price is usually warranted.

Fixed Assets

Medical equipment

In most transactions, all the medical equipment in the practice, large and small, is transferred to the buyer unless otherwise noted. The value of this equipment is usually agreed to by the buyer and seller. The value of this equipment is supposed to equate to FMV.

Office equipment/computer equipment/furniture and fixtures

In most transactions, all these assets are transferred unless otherwise noted. It is not uncommon for a seller to want to keep his old desk or a sentimental picture. It is customary for attorneys to identify these nontransferring items on a separate schedule within the asset-transferring contracts. Generally, all other assets are part of the sale. The allocated value is usually agreed to by the buyer and seller.

Leasehold improvements

If the buyer is buying a veterinary practice that is in a leased facility, the actual value of the practice's leasehold improvements (build-out of the space) may depend on a number of factors: the age and condition of these assets; the amount of time left on the lease; and the specific terms of the lease, such as whether the lessor or the lessee owns the actual leasehold improvements. If the buyer is buying a veterinary practice along with the building, the leasehold improvements are generally included in the value of the building he or she is buying. So, in general, although the leasehold improvements stay with the veterinary practice, their ownership and value may not. Be careful to specify whether equipment like surgical lights is included in equipment or in leasehold improvements. The same is true for built-in cabinets, which may be classified as equipment or may be part of the initial build-out of the space. Be sure these items do not get left out or duplicated.

Other Assets

Deposits

For a leased facility, a rent or security deposit may or may not be transferred with the practice, depending on the details of the transaction. Other deposits, such as for utilities, are generally not transferred.

Liabilities

Current liabilities/long-term liabilities

Generally speaking, in an asset sale, no existing liabilities are transferred to the buyer. All long-term debt, credit lines, credit cards payable, accounts payable, and accrued expenses are the responsibility of the seller. The buyer usually starts with a clean slate. The only debt he or she takes on is usually the amount borrowed to purchase the veterinary practice itself.

Equipment leases

Some equipment that is purchased by the buyer may have an existing lease attached to it. The current amount owed on this equipment lease should be factored into the overall value of the veterinary practice. Many equipment leases are transferable (only with the permission of the lessor) but are not assignable. In other words, the lease is transferable to the buyer, but the ultimate responsibility for payment of the lease remains with the original lessee (the seller).

Again, in general, the buyer of a veterinary practice can expect to purchase the existing clients of the practice (intangible assets) and the operational assets needed to service those clients properly (tangible assets).

Lack of Marketability: How This Influences Value

Two veterinary practices can have the same gross revenues, the same cash flow, the same great staff, and the same state-of-the-art equipment. They both go on the market on the same day for the same asking price. One sells, however, whereas as the other does not. Why?

Some veterinary practices, even high-quality ones, can suffer from a lack of marketability. This lack of marketability means that for one reason or another, the owner has difficulty in finding a buyer for the stated price. Usually, a lack of marketability can be attributed to one of two factors: location or specialization (niche).

The first of these factors to be considered is location. Veterinary practice owners in unpopulated, unusual, or difficult locations can find it hard to sell a practice. The pool of potential buyers is diminished greatly. A rural small animal practice in Montana, for instance, may do all the right things and have a tremendous cash flow, but if there are not a lot of buyers wanting to live in that specific location, the owner may have difficulty in selling it.

The second of these factors is specialization. A veterinary practice that has a specialization or a specific niche can find itself in the same situation. If a practice specializes in pocket pets, for instance, only buyers with an interest and a talent for pocket pets are going to desire this practice. Again, this limits the pool of potential buyers.

If not careful, appraisers of these types of veterinary practices can find a disconnection between their calculated value and what these practices actually end up selling for. To adjust for this, appraisers apply what is called a marketability discount. This is an amount deducted from the calculated value for a lack of marketability. For instance, a practice may have a calculated value of

$1,000,000; however, because of a perceived lack of marketability, the appraiser decides to apply a 10% marketability discount, making a final FMV determination of $900,000. Based on the appraiser's knowledge and experience, this $900,000 is more in line with what the veterinary practice is actually going to command on the open market.

For this group of practices, the theory is that more and more buyers might be willing to buy the practice at a lower price. The goal is to find where these two lines intersect. The marketability discount is not an exact science and is usually determined based on the experience of the appraiser. A marketability discount of 30% or 40% is not uncommon.

An owner with a veterinary practice that suffers from a lack of marketability needs to take steps early to deal with this. Finding an associate willing to buy in could be a way to secure the seller's eventual exit and still maintain the value of the practice. In other words, the practice may be worth more to an associate who already lives and works there rather than to a hypothetical buyer.

THE GREAT GIVEAWAY: COSTS OF SELLING A PORTION OF YOUR PRACTICE

Practice owners commonly find themselves faced with the dilemma of whether or not to sell a piece of their practice to an associate. The reasons to do so are often compelling. Selling part of a practice may be a means of ensuring that a superior associate stays in the practice, and it can also provide the owner(s) with a workable exit strategy and a willing buyer when that day arrives. Furthermore, it may be a way to shift part of the burden of ownership responsibilities to others. Finally, an associate can provide new or renewed enthusiasm to the practice's ownership and enable the practice to grow more rapidly in the future.

Although there may be significant reasons to sell to an associate, the decision to sell a portion of one's practice is not always fiscally sound for the seller. This article examines the underlying reasons why this is true. In most buy-in situations, the seller is at best giving a portion of the practice away, and in most buy-ins, significant financial losses are often incurred by the seller. To aid the reader in understanding this phenomenon, a rather typical buy-in scenario is presented. It is important for the reader to monitor the cash flows in the accompanying charts.

Common Scenario
Owner
Dr. Owner is an overworked practitioner who spends more hours at the practice than he would like. The demands of the practice have interfered with his participation in family activities. His practice is understaffed with veterinarians, and although he has been actively seeking an additional staff veterinarian, his efforts have been unsuccessful. He has thought:

> I do not see how anyone can keep a good associate veterinarian without making her part owner...

The only way she would come to work for me was with the promise that she could have ownership at some point in the future. She left another high-paying position because the owners of that practice would not offer her ownership. She is just too good to take the chance of losing her.

The practice is rapidly growing and with my valued associate sharing the ownership and responsibilities, I know we can increase the value of the practice many fold.

Associate

Dr. Associate has been employed by the practice for 3 years and is capable, intelligent, and well liked by the clients. Dr. Owner is concerned that she may decide to move on to a new practice and leave him severely understaffed and overworked. Dr. Associate graduated from veterinary school with approximately $110,000 in educational debt. She is married, and her husband has a fairly low-paying job in the community. They have two wonderful daughters. Approximately a year ago, they bought their first house, making a minimal down payment and financing the remainder over 30 years. In spite of Dr. Associate's wisely frugal nature, because of the cash flow requirements of the educational debt, the real estate mortgage, and the demands of everyday living, she and her husband have been able to save less than $15,000. Her parents plan to help her make a minimal down payment toward the purchase of a piece of the practice. She has inquired at her local bank and several others about the possibility of securing a loan for a partial practice acquisition. All have indicated that they are not willing to provide a practice acquisition loan unless they have a guarantor or the seller pledges all the practice assets toward the loan.

Promise

Ever since the original negotiations with the associate, Dr. Owner has indicated, implied, and promised that a partnership opportunity existed for the right individual. Recently, Dr. Associate has reminded him of his long-standing promise and has indicated that she would like to pursue this partnership opportunity in the near future.

Buy-in

In this example, the practice generates $700,000 in revenue and was recently valued for $560,000. Operating earnings (net profits after all normal operating expenses, including the owner's salary) are 15% of gross fees. Dr. Owner has decided to offer Dr. Associate 50% of the practice for $280,000. The terms of the transaction are summarized in Fig. 3.[c]

---

[c]The terms set forth in this scenario are somewhat idealized so as to facilitate the reader's understanding. Two examples of idealized assumptions follow: (1) the seller is willing to sell 50% of his practice, and (2) the buyer and seller are identically compensated for their veterinary services. These possible but unlikely assumptions neutralize the effect of their respective cash flows, thus facilitating the reader's ability to focus on those case flows specifically affected by the associate's buy-in. Also, for the same reason, all income taxes have been ignored, except as discussed below.

The Practice		
Revenue		700,000
Operating Earnings	15%	105,000
Value (as a % of revenue)	80%	560,000
Terms of Sale		
Percent sold		50%
Value of 50% ownership		280,000

Fig. 3. Terms of the transaction.

Because it is often difficult to obtain commercial funding for buy-ins, Dr. Owner has agreed to hold the note for Dr. Associate. Fig. 4 summarizes the loan terms.

Before the buy-in, both doctors were producing at similar levels and both were compensated at 22% of their production. Thus, both doctors were receiving the same compensation for their veterinary efforts. Dr. Seller, as owner, also received the practice profits. The cash flow to each doctor in year 1 is shown in Fig. 5.

Dr. Associate now has to make payments on her loan to Dr. Seller for the buy-in. The cash flows now look as in Fig. 6.

In particular, compare Dr. Associate's cash flow in Figs. 5 and 6. Both doctors received the same compensation and earnings distributions. The cash flow she now receives from her share of the profits approximates her loan payments to Dr. Seller. On the surface, it seems that Dr. Owner and Dr. Associate's positions before and after buy-in have remained much the same. The money has essentially gone in a circle, with each doctor's financial position relatively unchanged even though the buyer paid taxes on her salary and her share of the profits, with only the interest portion of the payments being deductible to her, at best. The seller also paid taxes on the principal and interest portions of the payments he received from her. After the buy-in, Dr. Owner is still bringing home approximately $180,000 a year for the first 7 years and Dr. Associate continues to receive slightly less than $80,000. On a year-to-year basis, each doctor's financial situation seems to be much the same as before the buy-in, except for the income tax effect.

Terms of Loan		
Holder of the Loan		Dr. Owner
Price 50%		280,000
Down payment	5%	14,000
Loan amount		266,000
Interest rate		9%
Term in years		7
Payment / month		4,280
Payment / annual		51,356

Fig. 4. Terms of the loan.

	Owner	Associate
Production Percent Compensation	50%	50%
Doctor's Revenue Production	350,000	350,000
Percent Compensation	22%	22%
Compensation	77,000	77,000
Practice earnings	105,000	-
Total Cash Flow from Practice	182,000	77,000

Fig. 5. Cash flows if no buy-in (year 1).

When the annual cash flows are accumulated over the 7 years of the entire transaction, however, they are much changed. To illustrate this, first look at Fig. 7, which summarizes each of the 7 years of the proposed buy-in. In this case, however, the buy-in does not take place (ie, Dr. Seller continues to own 100% of the practice). This illustration serves as a baseline to compare the effects of the buy-in transaction on the buyer and the seller. In particular, in the "Totals" column at the right, note that although the compensation to both doctors is the same, Dr. Owner has more than $2.2 million of cumulative cash inflows, including his salary, the profits, and the estimated equity value of the practice at the end of the 7-year period (estimated at 80% of revenue). The illustration clearly shows the wide variation in cash flow as a result of Dr. Owner retaining 100% ownership.

Fig. 8 illustrates the cash flows for a 7-year period as in Fig. 7; however, in this scenario, Dr. Associate has purchased 50% of the practice. The "Total" column sums the 7-year cumulative cash flows in this transaction as follows: (1) cumulative compensation for work as a veterinarian and (2) repayment of the buy-in loan. In addition, each owner's equity value at the end of the transaction (end of the seventh year) is shown.

Fig. 9 summarizes the data shown in Figs. 7 and 8. The two columns on the left provide the cumulative cash flows in the no buy-in circumstance. The two columns on the right show the cumulative cash flows in the buy-in circumstance. In addition, each doctor's estimated equity value at the end of the 7 years is shown.

		Owner	Associate
Production Percent Compensation		50%	50%
Dr. Revenue Production		350,000	350,000
Percent Compensation		22%	22%
Compensation		77,000	77,000
Practice earnings	50%	52,500	52,500
Total Cash Flow from Practice		129,500	129,500
Dr. Associate's Loan Payment		51,356	(51,356)
Cash flows after Buy-in Year 1		180,856	78,144

Fig. 6. Cash flows after the buy-in (year 1).

CASH FLOWS IF NO SALE								
	1	2	3	4	5	6	7	Total
Revenue (5% annual grow	700,000	735,000	771,750	810,338	850,854	893,397	938,067	
Profits (15% revenue)	105,000	110,250	115,763	121,551	127,628	134,010	140,710	
Dr. Owner								
Compensation	77,000	80,850	84,893	89,137	93,594	98,274	103,187	626,935
Profits (15% revenue)	105,000	110,250	115,763	121,551	127,628	134,010	140,710	854,911
Cash flow to Owner	182,000	191,100	200,655	210,688	221,222	232,283	243,897	1,481,846
Equity Value of Practice 80% Rev.								750,454
Total of 7 yr Cash Flows + Equity Value								2,232,299
Dr. Associate								
Compensation	77,000	80,850	84,893	89,137	93,594	98,274	103,187	626,935
Profits (15% revenue)	-	-	-	-	-	-	-	
Cash flow to Associate	77,000	80,850	84,893	89,137	93,594	98,274	103,187	626,935

Fig. 7. Cumulative cash flows over the 7-year period, with no sale to the associate.

What has happened to Dr. Seller?

In return for selling a 50% ownership interest in the practice to Dr. Associate over a 7-year period, Dr. Owner gains $373,494 from the 50% sale (down payment, loan principle, and interest) but loses $427,455 in cumulative profits and has given up $375,227 in equity value at the end of year 7. In summary, at the end of 7 years, Dr. Owner has a net loss of $429,188.

What has happened to Dr. Associate?

Dr. Associate, by buying a 50% ownership in the practice over a 7-year period, pays out $373,494 for the 50% buy-in (down payment, principle, and interest), gains $427,455 in cumulative profits, and has gained $375,227 in equity value at the end of the year 7. In summary, at the end of 7 years, Dr. Associate has a net gain of $429,188.

Four Important Observations

Circular flow of cash

During the buy-in, Dr. Owner's money essentially goes in a circle. For this observation, compare the three cumulative cash flows in Fig. 9. The

CASH FLOWS AFTER SALE	Years of the Buy-In Loan Repayment							
	1	2	3	4	5	6	7	Total
Revenue	700,000	735,000	771,750	810,338	850,854	893,397	938,067	
Profits (15% revenue)	105,000	110,250	115,763	121,551	127,628	134,010	140,710	
Dr. Owner								
Compensation	77,000	80,850	84,893	89,137	93,594	98,274	103,187	626,935
Profits (15% revenue)	52,500	55,125	57,881	60,775	63,814	67,005	70,355	427,455
CF from operations	129,500	135,975	142,774	149,912	157,408	165,278	173,542	1,054,390
Loan inflows 14,000	51,356	51,356	51,356	51,356	51,356	51,356	51,356	373,494
Cash flows to Owner	180,856	187,331	194,130	201,269	208,764	216,635	224,899	1,427,884
Equity Value of Practice 80% Rev.								375,227
Total of 7 yr Cash Flows + Equity Value								1,803,111
Dr. Associate								
Compensation	77,000	80,850	84,893	89,137	93,594	98,274	103,187	626,935
Profits (15% revenue)	52,500	55,125	57,881	60,775	63,814	67,005	70,355	427,455
CF from operations	129,500	135,975	142,774	149,912	157,408	165,278	173,542	1,054,390
Loan outflows #######	(51,356)	(51,356)	(51,356)	(51,356)	(51,356)	(51,356)	(51,356)	(373,494)
Cash flows to Assoc	78,144	84,619	91,417	98,556	106,052	113,922	122,186	680,896
Equity Value of Practice 80% Rev.								375,227
Total of 7 yr Cash Flows + Equity Value								1,056,123

Fig. 8. Cash flows over the 7 years of the transaction (50%).

SUMMARY OF CASH FLOWS +EST. PRACTICE VALUE AT END OF YEAR 7				
		End of First 7 Years		
		No Buy-In		50% Buy-In	
		Owner	Associate	Owner	Associate
CF1	Cumulative compensation	626,935	626,935	626,935	626,935
CF2	Cumulative profits to each owner	854,911	-	427,455	427,455
CF3	Cumulative 7 years loan Pmts.	-	-	373,494	(373,494)
CF total	Subtotal of cash flows	1,481,846	626,935	1,427,884	680,896
Equity	Practice Value End Year 7 (80% Rev.)	750,454		375,227	375,227
	Cumulative cash flow	2,232,299	626,935	1,803,111	1,056,123

Fig. 9. Summary of cash flows.

compensation cash flow (CF1) is not affected by the change in ownership. The distribution of earnings (CF2) shows that 50% of the earnings are now shifted to Dr. Associate as a result of her 50% buy-in. Dr. Associate now repays a similar amount back to Dr. Owner as part of the debt repayment (CF3). Thus, Dr. Owner's money has moved in a circle.

Most sellers do not perceive the potential losses they are incurring because they do not understand the impact of the buy-in at the end of 7 years
During the 7 years of the transaction, neither the associate nor the seller sees much change in annual cash flow from the ownership changes, ignoring the income tax effect to each. As discussed in observation 1, by just examining cash flows, taking an associate into an ownership position would seem to be an approximately break-even situation.

Change in ownership equity
Because the change in equity or ownership value is not usually considered a cash flow, it is often overlooked as a cost of taking in an associate as a partner. The effect on ownership worth is always negative, at least initially, because the seller now owns less of the practice than previously. In the ideal circumstance, the new partner helps to create a significant increase in the worth of the practice. If the two owners together can grow the practice and increase its value more than in this example, the loss to the seller can then be more than offset by this increase in practice value. Unfortunately, in most buy-ins, the increase in practice worth does not outpace the equity loss to the owner incurred by the transfer of ownership. Unless the seller maintains partial ownership for many years after the buy-in, there is likely not enough time to recoup the losses described previously.

Changes in cash flows after the debt repayment
As discussed, neither Dr. Seller nor Dr. Associate is likely to perceive any change in total cash flow during the loan repayment years. Fig. 10 shows cash flows coming to the associate and the seller over the 7 years of the transaction and 2 years beyond. During the initial 7 years, the difference between the seller's cash flow and the associate's cash flow is the loan repayment funds. In year 7, the loan is paid off. Immediately thereafter, Dr. Seller experiences a significant drop in cash flow, and Dr. Associate experiences a significant increase.

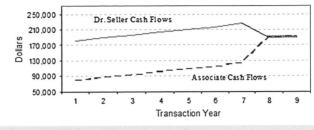

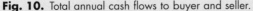

Fig. 10. Total annual cash flows to buyer and seller.

Concluding Thoughts

The purpose of this article is not to discourage practice owners from selling a portion of their practice to an associate. Rather, the purpose is to educate owners to the potential costs associated with a partial sale and that these costs may be significantly greater than initially perceived. Too often, practice owners enter into partnerships with associates without any consideration of the financial costs incurred.

There are, of course, many sound reasons for bringing an associate into ownership:

- Associate ownership may be a part of a well-developed exit strategy. If the seller plans to sell the remainder of the practice within a couple of years, the impact on the seller's long-term cash flow is largely irrelevant. The seller does not plan to remain in practice ownership and share in the profits anyway.
- Associate ownership may be justified as a means of retaining an exceptional associate who, without an ownership offer, might seek other employment.
- Associate ownership may be a part of a strategy to reduce and share the non-veterinary work and time obligations associated with ownership (ie, general practice management, personnel problems).

The assumptions used in this discussion to illustrate and emphasize major cash flows may paint a discouraging picture. In most cases, associates are not sold 50% of the practice, they do not produce at the same level as the owner, and they are not paid the same as the owner. There are sound strategies to reduce the seller's potential losses and still provide for the associate's needs. These strategies include the following:

- Limiting the percentage of the practice to be sold to the associate. Owners can significantly reduce the financial impact by limiting the initial ownership transfer to 20% or less. If the point is to ensure a buyer for the rest of the practice when the seller exits, there is no need to sell a large portion now.
- Significantly increasing the compensation paid to the associate while delaying a transfer of ownership. This may be an attractive alternative to ownership for some associates.
- Entering into an agreement that provides the associate with an option to buy at some future date

- Restructuring the transaction so that less income tax is paid on the practice's profits before they reach the seller during the buy-in period (ie, a compensation shift)
- Customizing the buy-in to include a combination of these strategies

C CORPORATION ISSUES AND HOW THIS MAY INFLUENCE VALUE

As mentioned previously, more than 90% of veterinary practice sale transactions are structured as asset sales. For reasons discussed later in this article, buyers of practices rarely buy stock. Of the few stock transactions occurring, most occur in associate partial buy-ins to an existing practice operating as a corporation. In these buy-in cases, the buyer who is purchasing only a piece of a practice necessarily buys the practice as it is currently structured, which may mean buying shares of stock. Many sellers today, especially those approaching retirement, find themselves in a tough situation: in the process of preparing their practice for a future sale, these owners are discovering that their C (regular) corporations, once useful and powerful tools for tax purposes, are now incredible financial and tax burdens because of double taxation. The double taxation of C corporations comes about when the corporation sells its assets rather than the shareholder selling his or her stock. Because there are generally no buyers willing to purchase stock, the owner of the corporate practice is forced to sell the assets within the corporation instead. By selling the practice assets, the seller is faced with an initial tax at the corporate level—income tax levied on the gain from the sale of the practice (corporate) assets. Then, a second tax is levied at the personal level—income tax assessed on the net after-tax proceeds realized from sale of the corporation and paid to the seller individually. That is an incredible price to pay, and it is not unusual to see between 50% and 60% of the sales proceeds going to the government.

Why the preference for assets over stock? For one, many assets can be depreciated or amortized for tax purposes, whereas stock in a corporation cannot. An asset purchase provides valuable tax deductions for a buyer with a tight cash flow. In general, the tangible assets that are purchased (eg, medical equipment, computer equipment, fixtures) can be depreciated over 5 to 7 years. Intangible assets purchased (eg, goodwill, patient records, covenant not to compete) can be amortized over 15 years.

A buyer who purchases stock must hold that stock and hope that he or she can recoup the lost tax benefits when the new practice is eventually sold. That is a long time to wait for valuable tax deductions. Because of these tax burdens, the fact is that there are few buyers out there willing to pay full price for shares in a C corporation. As a result, the seller really only has two options, neither of which is attractive: sell the stock of his or her veterinary corporation at a severely discounted price and take the financial hit or sell the practice assets, deal with the double taxation of his corporation, and take the financial hit.

Another reason to avoid a stock purchase is corporate baggage. When someone buys a corporation, the purchaser is also buying the corporation's history and all the corporation's existing and potential problems. Internal Revenue Service (IRS) audits, back sales tax owed, and former employee issues, for example, all become the responsibility of the current owner. Buying a corporation that has been alive for 20 years means 20 years of history for which the buyer takes responsibility. The sales contract can indemnify the buyer and try to hold the seller responsible; however, at a minimum, the buyer does get pulled into the fray because of being the current owner.

During negotiations, a veterinarian owning a C corporation naturally prefers the opposite perspective of the buyer: the seller always wants to sell his or her stock, whereas the buyer always wants to buy assets.

What can the owners of C corporations do to avoid this problem? With proper tax planning and enough lead time, they can turn their C corporation into an S corporation. An S corporation is a "flow-through" type of entity, meaning that in most situations, no tax is paid at the corporate level. All the income generated by the S corporation "flows through" to the shareholder. The election is relatively painless and, once in effect, allows the seller to sidestep double taxation. A major caveat exists, however: there is a 10-year period before the election fully takes effect, so proper planning is required. Otherwise, if a sale of corporate assets occurs before the 10-year window is up, the sale of assets is basically treated for tax purposes as though the S corporation election had never been made (ie, double taxation).

So, although the C corporation situation may not affect the appraised value of a veterinary practice, it does have an impact on the seller's eventual cash flow. This affects what he or she is willing to sell the practice for, because the after-tax proceeds are much smaller than the sales price.

So, what can be done for sellers who are in this position? Usually, they have two options. First, they can discount the price of the practice enough to make it worth the buyer's while. What is that discount? It is difficult to say, because the discount can vary depending on the total purchase price and the buyer's individual situation.

Second, they can try to negotiate an asset allocation that provides them some favorable tax treatment. Certain assets of the practice can perhaps be sold outside of the corporation, such as the covenant not to compete, personal goodwill, or a consulting agreement. Structuring this correctly can be tricky, so please consult with your experienced certified public accountant (CPA).

Like the marketability discount, sellers in this predicament have to offer major concessions (eg, price discounts, creative financing) to sell the practice and gain the most cash flow possible.

References

[1] McCafferty OE. How to price your practice. Veterinary Economics 1987; Aug: 38–55.
[2] McCafferty OE. How to price your practice. Veterinary Economics 1987; Sep: 62–71.
[3] McCafferty OE. How to price your practice. Veterinary Economics 1987; Oct: 62–9.

Vet Clin Small Anim 36 (2006) 329–339

VETERINARY CLINICS
SMALL ANIMAL PRACTICE

The Gender Shift in Veterinary Medicine: Cause and Effect

Carin A. Smith, DVM*

Smith Veterinary Consulting, PO Box 698, Peshastin, WA 98847, USA

A great deal of discussion, speculation, and study has focused on the dramatic increase in women veterinarians. Much of the gender discussion revolves around economics and business management. In veterinary medicine, great concerns about debt and income have arisen at the same time that the number of women in practice has increased. It is crucial to avoid making assumptions about cause and effect when several changes happen concurrently.

When discussing gender and work, one must first gain a historical perspective about women in the workplace. Then, a look at changes in veterinary medicine can give information about this profession. Finally, one can examine studies of men, women, and work, both within and outside the veterinary profession. That approach will give information about current issues and ideas for action steps to improve the profession for all.

WOMEN AND WORK IN THE UNITED STATES

Much of the change in women working results from economic conditions and from the equal opportunity laws enacted in the 1970s [1]. Those changes, however, are not sufficient to explain the dramatic increase of women in only certain professions.

It is easy to focus on certain job attributes that are stereotypically female and that would "make" women "good at" or "suitable for" particular professions. Research, however, shows that these factors are used as after-the-fact explanations that do not thoroughly explain women's increased entry into some professions. For instance, one might focus on the human–animal bond and thus say that a stereotypically nurturing woman would be a "good" veterinarian. One could also focus on the increasingly complex surgical, computerized, and technical aspects of veterinary medicine to explain why a stereotypical man would make a "good" veterinarian [2,3].

*Correspondence. PO Box 698, Peshastin, WA 98847. E-mail address:
info@smithvet.com

0195-5616/06/$ – see front matter
doi:10.1016/j.cvsm.2005.11.001

An in-depth analysis was done of a wide variety of professions, over several decades, whose members changed from predominantly men to predominantly women (a greater increase of women than was seen in the overall workforce). This study revealed that all the professions studied underwent a decline in job prestige or real earnings. In most of these jobs (including pharmacy, editing/reporting, and bank management), status and pay had already dropped before women's rapid entry [2].

WOMEN AND MEN IN VETERINARY MEDICINE

The question of whether women's entry into the profession "caused" the current economic concerns in veterinary medicine is easily answered by looking at enrollment and income data. The number of male applicants (and total applicants) declined between 1981 and 1990. The data show that the drop in male applicants followed a decreased demand for large-animal veterinarians and a decrease in real income. Thereafter the total number of applicants rose, but male applicant numbers remained low. A reduction in male applicants has fueled the increase in female veterinarians (KPMG analysis, unpublished chart derived from American Association of Veterinary Medical Colleges data) [4].

One might ask whether the male veterinarians of the past actually "caused" the income problem, but a narrow focus on gender or on blame misses the larger economic changes that have occurred during the past 30 to 50 years. Whatever the cause, the current situation is of concern because of the high debt-to-income ratio of today's veterinary school graduates.

Along with the economic drivers of the gender shift, of course, is the simple fact that women do want to become veterinarians. Lost in the discussion is why fewer men may want to do so. It seems that financial considerations are a driving force.

IS IT GENERATION OR GENDER?

Is the income problem one of gender or simply one of different lifestyle choices made by the new generation? Are the changing attitudes toward work an attribute of the generation and not limited to women? It is true that younger generations of men do express more interest in family, in working fewer hours, and in balancing their lives between work and other activities. The true test, though, is in research studies that track the actual time that men and women spend with career and family, not the amount of time they plan to spend or wish they could spend.

DVM Newsmagazine reported that more men than women complained they worked too many hours. That complaint does not lead to a difference in actual hours worked by men. Although women with children spent less time at work than those without children, men with children spent slightly more time at work than did men without children (when men say "family is important," that statement translates into working more). In fact, single women (without children) worked the same number of hours as did men with children [5].

A vast amount of research shows that this trend holds true for women in a wide variety of professions. One study of women physicians found that only 49% of women with children had achieved their career goals, compared with 80% of women without children and 78% of men with children [6].

Much media attention has focused on shifting gender roles in the household, but there is little or no direct evidence that these changes are significant. A study of "Gen X" fathers showed they spent more hours per week at work than employees of comparable ages in 1977 [7]. Research shows that women still do 80% of childcare and two thirds of housework. Being a home manager takes time and energy that is not recognized by most couples (the father helps, but first the mother figures out what he needs to do) [8].

Women and Time

Because there are a finite number of hours in the day, simple math shows that women do not have the same amount of time to devote to business matters as do men. Women who do want to work full time are often frustrated or suffer from burnout from competing demands [9]. If women want to earn more, and they are already as productive as men on an hourly basis, their next choice is to work more hours. If women want to participate more in organized veterinary medicine, they need to create more free hours. One way to get those extra hours is for husbands and fathers take on more of the "home work" to free up women's time. Thus, women need both more business knowledge and the ability and skills to negotiate for equity in their home lives.

On the other hand, many women choose to work part time. These veterinarians are fulfilling their personal goals and are also filling an important niche in veterinary medicine. Many hospitals do not need or cannot afford a full-time second or third veterinarian, and many women are eager to fill this void. Unfortunately, part-time veterinarians are often held in little esteem, considered less dedicated, or left out of the loop with regard to practice communications [10]. The profession needs a change in attitude to recognize the value of part-time veterinarians. In turn, part-timers must recognize the tradeoffs they make when choosing not to work full time.

EFFECTS OF PART TIME OR TIME OUT ON CAREER PATH

The tendency of mothers to work part time or to take time out has implications on the career paths of women as compared with men. One study of women physicians done 10 years after their medical school graduation showed that one third of them had taken a maternity/child care leave, and 24% had taken time away from their careers for other reasons, compared with 11% of men who had interrupted their careers. If this trend holds true for veterinarians, women may reach career milestones such as practice ownership at a later age than do men [11].

A study of women physicians showed that the hours worked by full-time and part-time women did not correlate with their career satisfaction. Overall, both part-timers and full-timers were equally satisfied with their careers. Marital quality did not affect the career satisfaction of full-time women physicians, but women physicians who worked part time and also had unsatisfactory marriages were much more likely to report that they considered dropping out of the profession [12].

Having a child has a significant negative effect on a woman's income. The "motherhood penalty" is a common explanation for women's lower incomes. Women exit the labor market more often than do men. The result is said to be slower advancement or atrophy of skills or knowledge.

Several studies have examined the motherhood wage gap. The gap between non-mothers and mothers is between 7% and 16% for one child and 29% for two or more children. The highest total penalty is borne by college-educated mothers of two or more children. (The penalty for one child is much less than one half of the penalty for two or more.) Some studies found that the wage gap was explained by years out of the workforce (the "human capital" explanation), whereas others found that only about one third of the gap could be explained by less work experience or atrophy of skills. It is possible that employer perceptions and assumptions about these women's skills could have an effect [13–15].

MEN, WOMEN, AND PRACTICE OWNERSHIP

It is a myth that women do not want to own practices. In fact, female students state they do want to become owners, but the expressed interest wanes after graduation. In spite of that expressed disinterest, however, women are buying practices. *DVM Newsmagazine* reported that about half of female veterinarian associates expressed an interest in practice ownership, contrary to fears otherwise [16]. Simmons Associates, a practice brokerage firm, reported that 39% of all transactions are to women, with the number rising continually. A small survey of consultants revealed that 47% of all their practice sales involved women [17].

Several factors seem to be at work. First, self-reporting of one's future intentions is often misleading. Next, because of childbearing responsibilities, women may become owners on a different life-timeline than do men. And finally, women face the challenge of learning about and developing flexible working arrangements to allow them to meet other demands and responsibilities. With creative thought and planning, men and women do not have to repeat the old model of overwork and burnout as practice owners.

MEN, WOMEN, AND RURAL OR LARGE-ANIMAL PRACTICE

Much speculation and discussion have revolved around the association between the increased number of women in the profession and the shortage of large-animal veterinarians.

First, it is necessary to define terms. A rural practice is often a mixed practice or, if it is a large-animal practice, services small farms. In contrast, the new large-animal veterinarian is a consultant who works with one or more very large livestock producers.

The loudest concerns about a shortage of large-animal veterinarians seem to originate from rural veterinarians. If one asks any rural veterinary practitioners about whether they need new associate veterinarians, the answer is likely to be "yes." They often express concern about whether anyone will want to buy their practices.

Are these concerns real evidence that there is a shortage? From a strictly economic viewpoint, economic benefit should follow a high demand for these services. One of the biggest obstacles to getting veterinarians to work in rural areas, however, is the low pay in proportion to the hours worked. To be able to serve a rural area—to be available at all hours as needed, but to serve a very small total population—means that the income per hour is going to be low.

Care must be taken to avoid the assumption that attracting men from rural backgrounds will fill the need for rural veterinarians. Even if this effort were successful, would those young graduates turn to urban small-animal practice, just to pay their debts?

In reading about the shortage of associate veterinarians, almost all of the opinions come from the demand side (employers). Many veterinary students express interest in rural or mixed practice but end up working in urban or suburban small-animal practices. Instead of asking employers in rural areas why they cannot find someone to fill their job, one might better ask potential employees why they do not take up those offers. After all, they are the ones making the decision, so they probably know the reason.

Home and lifestyle factors, in addition to economic factors, affect the types and locations of jobs chosen by women. Although it is tempting to blame their background or to assume simplistically that women do not like large animal practice, no data support those suppositions.

Almost half of female physicians who do work in rural areas were not raised in rural environments, but most planned to stay where they worked. Female physicians report that their decision to work in a rural area depends on whether their spouse can get a job, as well as on lifestyle factors such as flexible scheduling and availability of child care [18–21].

Perhaps part of the problem in filling rural veterinarian positions is inadequate job choice for spouses in rural areas or the lower income of mixed animal practices, so that school debt cannot be repaid. Also, women's home obligations make it impossible for them to work the same number of hours as did the previous generation of men who had full-time, stay-at-home wives.

Rural practitioners who seek new associates might be more successful recruiting for two part-time positions than in looking for one person who will work those longer hours. They also might consider offering assistance in spousal job placement. Finally, thoughtful questioning of those who turn down rural jobs might reveal more complex answers than the oversimplified scapegoats of location or income alone.

CURRENT FINANCIAL STATUS OF MEN AND WOMEN VETERINARIANS

Several recent studies highlight new and sometimes conflicting information about income and gender. Each also leaves some open questions or unknown areas that need further evaluation. Contrary to what some headlines would state, it is not impossible to find out more information, and there are not too many variables to consider. Further analysis will require complex thinking and higher-level investigation. For example, owner income data are hard to compare, because many owners have different business entities, different bonus systems, and different ways of paying profits.

American Veterinary Medical Association Data

The American Veterinary Medical Association (AVMA) data showed that women veterinarians earn less than do men. This difference held true when the data were stratified by associates versus owners, by years out of practice, and by type of practice. The report still left open some questions, including whether differences in practice owner incomes result from age (of the veterinarian and of the practice) or gender alone [22].

The AVMA found that veterinarians' incomes are increasing, but that mean income for male veterinarians increased faster than that for women. Practice ownership, gender, community size, and employee development were the variables with the strongest relationship to personal income [23].

As of 2003, 19% of female veterinarians worked less than 30 hours per week. Women earned less than men even when they worked the same number of hours, had similar years of experience, and when comparisons were made among just associates or just owners [22].

Men scored higher than women in financial concepts. Women scored higher than men in leadership. Both items are correlated with higher income [22].

The length of time that a practice had been in operation differed between men and women owners. Women owners earned less than men owners, but women owners' practices had been in business a mean of 18 years, whereas men's practices had been in business a mean of 28 years [22].

The summary report listed specific items that are correlated with higher income. Improving these factors can improve the income of any individual. Although there was no evidence that veterinarians are using more of the best business practices, their income from 1997 to 2003 rose nonetheless. The main influence was raising fees, because almost all respondents indicated they had done so, with fewer pointing to practice growth or reducing expenses as influencers [22].

American Animal Hospital Association Data

The American Animal Hospital Association (AAHA) evaluated several factors that affect income. Both AAHA and non-AAHA practices were surveyed. Of the variables analyzed, practice ownership explained the highest degree of variation in veterinarians' salaries [24].

When practice owners were evaluated, male practice owners earned more than female practice owners. Men reported being in their current position significantly longer than women, which may explain some of the difference in earnings. The study answered several other questions that had not been previously evaluated [23].

Among practice owners, all the following items do affect income. Gender differences in income were not caused by any of these factors [23]:

- Hours worked per week did not differ by gender (average, 49 hours)
- More full time equivalent (FTE) veterinarians in practice led to higher incomes. Men and women were equally likely to work in practices with the same number of FTEs.
- Sole owners had a higher income per owner than did multiple owners, but men and women were equally likely to work alone as with other owners.
- Veterinarians in exclusively small-animal practices earn more than those in mixed practice. Men and women were equally likely to work in either type of practice.
- Neighborhood income affects income, but men and women were distributed equally.
- Region of the country affects income, but men and women were distributed equally.
- Board certification affects income, but men and women were equally likely to be certified.

Among associate veterinarians, the following items affect income [23]:

- The average salary paid and the average number of years male and female associate veterinarians were in their current positions were the same.
- Even though incomes were similar, the number of hours worked by female associates was significantly less (43) than their male peers (44.8). Possible explanations are that female associates are more likely than men to work in predominantly small-animal practices, which pay more, or perhaps women are more productive per hour.
- Information about total compensation, including benefits and bonuses, with gender comparisons was not offered.

DVM Newsmagazine Data

Several items of interest, in addition to those previously discussed, were revealed by *DVM Newsmagazine* surveys.

In contrast to the stereotype of women being more people-oriented, when asked what they enjoyed most about work, most men said "interacting with clients," whereas most women said "medical workups." Although both tended to enjoy client interaction more as they grew older, the gap remained through all ages, with more women than men saying that medical workups were most interesting [15].

Both men and women wanted to work fewer hours. Results stating what they want versus what they do are important signals of lifestyle and societal pressures. Men still spend more hours at work than women do [5].

The survey asked veterinarians how they feel about their personal financial situations. Among owners, fewer women (38%) than men (43%) feel their financial situation is satisfactory. Among associates, fewer men (28%) than women (31%) feel they have a satisfactory financial situation. Far more striking than those minor gender differences is the fact that less than half of men or women in any position felt they were earning enough. A vast majority of both said their main concern was about retirement [25].

Fifteen percent of men and 32% of women obtain health insurance through their spouse's employer [24]. Information about total compensation, including benefits and bonuses, with gender comparisons was not offered. Are women realizing that they should negotiate for higher pay in lieu of benefits they turn down?

STUDIES ABOUT WOMEN, WORK, PAY, AND SATISFACTION
Expectations, Satisfaction, Self-Assessment, and Self-Pay

Several studies both within veterinary medicine and from other professions have asked women whether they are "satisfied" with their income and have reported that women are satisfied with lower incomes than are men. What makes people "satisfied"? Is "satisfaction" a reliable measure of equality?

Research shows that people continually paid less than others for the same work will come to feel they are doing less than others and so are entitled to less pay. People who feel entitled to less ask for less and receive less. Expectations create reality. People asked to assign a salary will assign a higher salary to applicants who expect more money [3,26].

How many veterinary students are told, "You won't make money in this profession," or "Your clients won't pay for that"? Behavior follows expectations for both men and women in veterinary medicine.

Individuals prefer to compare themselves with people like themselves; this comparison preserves self-esteem and reduces feelings of deprivation. People also compare their current situation with their past situation. Women may expect lower pay because they have always received lower pay. Likewise, veterinarians may expect to not earn much because they have always been told they will not earn much. Thus, feeling good or being satisfied is not an accurate assessment of fair pay [25,27].

Men and women differ in their self-assessment and self-pay when doing the same work. When allowed to pay themselves, men overvalue and women undervalue their work. When working for the same amount of money, women work harder and longer than men do. Men rate their performance higher than do women when the same result is achieved [26].

There are many dangers to self-assessment. Surveys that ask respondents to self-assess their level of knowledge may inaccurately show women as less knowledgeable. Job interviewers who ask employees to self-assess their skills may get higher reports from men than from women. Self-evaluation in performance reviews may be skewed toward higher evaluation by males, and in negotiations for salary female veterinarians may underrate their worth. Self-evaluation can be valuable only if individuals are compared against their own prior self-evaluation—but never against others' self-evaluations.

The aforementioned studies were of people making decisions in the absence of outside information. Information reduces or eliminates gender differences.

When men or women are told what the average pay is for the work they are doing, they use that information to set pay for themselves, with no gender differences. When told they performed well, both men and women thought they deserved more money, with no gender differences in the amount.

When people learn that they are entitled to receive more than they do, the result is depression or anger, but ultimately change. The veterinary profession's response to the results of recent economic studies shows this reaction is occurring.

Professions that are primarily female now have a new challenge. How can one compare incomes to those of "similar males"? The answer is found in other studies of women and work. Instead of comparing "exact" jobs, one might compare "equivalent" jobs. For instance, one might compare housecleaners (primarily women) with janitors (primarily men) and look for any income differences. Likewise, veterinarians might compare themselves with other health care workers with a similar education.

IMPACT OF CONFUSING CAUSE AND EFFECT

The increased number of women in veterinary medicine has paralleled many other changes. It is crucial not to attribute cause-and-effect relationships unless those are proven. Cause and effect are often inadvertently confused. Note the differences in the following phrases, and what they assume about cause and effect:

- "Empathy causes women to earn less," versus "Earning less creates greater empathy."
- "Women's expectations cause them to earn less," versus "A history of earning less causes women to expect less."

Assumptions made about cause-and-effect relationships may lead to ineffective actions or policies. If the assumptions are not correct, the solution will not give the desired result.

If women earn less because they are inherently empathetic or have low self-esteem, then the cause lies in their personality, and an answer might be, "Gee, too bad, women will always just earn less, but they sure are nice!"

Which came first, high empathy, low self-esteem, or low income? Research shows that both men and women develop low self-esteem and develop higher empathy when they are in jobs that have low prestige, low pay, and low opportunity for advancement [28]. Improvement of skills, accurate positive performance evaluation, and a gain in income will increase their self-esteem. Furthermore, empathy and income need not be tradeoffs or exclusive of one another. It is not necessary for women to give up their empathy to charge fairly and to receive adequate compensation.

SUMMARY

Major strides have been made in collecting information that will help in understanding better the causes and effects of the increased number of women in the profession. To improve the profession's economic situation, veterinarians must share information about incomes (appropriately stratified), salaries (including the value of benefits), the basis of setting fees charged to clients, and what pet owners are willing to pay. Ask for and give accurate, objective, measurable performance feedback in the workplace.

Women's status in society is still undergoing dramatic change. In fact, some research shows that previously reported cognitive gender differences disappeared over several decades in parallel with women's changing position in society and education [29,30]. Today's young woman is far better equipped to enter the workforce than were prior generations. With awareness and open discussion of economic issues, it is possible to take positive steps for improvement. Recognize the complexities of gender and economics, and avoid falling back on oversimplified popular psychology. Complex problems have complex solutions; there is no single answer to the question of how gender and economics are tied together. Many clear steps, however, can be taken based on what the existing literature tells about men, women, and work.

References

[1] Bergman B. The economic emergence of women. New York: Basic Books; 1986. p. 19–27.
[2] Reskin B, Roos P. Job queues, gender queues. Explaining women's inroads into male occupations. Philadelphia: Temple University Press; 1990.
[3] Valian V. Why so slow? The advancement of women. Cambridge (MA): The MIT Press; 1998.
[4] The American Veterinary Medical Association, KPMG. The current and future market for veterinarians and veterinary services in the United States, 1999. Section II: emerging trends and markets, part 15.2, p. 104, 114.
[5] Verdon D. Work/life balance remains manageable, DVM survey says. DVM Newsmagazine 2004;16–21.
[6] Osler K. Employment experiences of vocationally trained doctors. BMJ 1991;303:762–4.
[7] Families and Work Institute. An analysis of the Generation and Gender in the Workplace Study published by the American Business Collaboration Oct 5, 2004. Available at: http://familiesandwork.org. Accessed June 19, 2005.
[8] Robinson J, Godbey G. Time for life: the surprising ways Americans use their time. University Park (PA): Penn State Press; 1999. p. 97–109.
[9] Linzer M, McMurray JE, Visser MR, et al. Sex differences in physician burnout in the US and The Netherlands. J Am Med Womens Assoc 2002;57(4):191–3.
[10] Littlewood J, Beer N, Lazou E, et al. Against women: are we looking after our general practitioners? GPs' views of the 1990 part-time contract. J R Soc Health 1999;119(2):85–8.
[11] Woodward CA, Cohen ML, Ferrier BM. Career interruptions and hours practiced: comparison between young men and women physicians. Can J Public Health 1990;81(1):16–20.
[12] Carr PL, Gareis KC, Barnett RC. Characteristics and outcomes for women physicians who work reduced hours. J Womens Health (Larchmt) 2003;12(4):399–405.
[13] Hewlett SA, Luce CB. Off-ramps and on-ramps: keeping talented women on the road to success. Harv Bus Rev 2005;83(3):43–6, 48, 50–4.
[14] Anderson D, et al. The motherhood wage penalty: who pays it, and why? Am Econ Rev 2002;92(2):354–8.
[15] Hotchkiss J, Pitts M. Maternity and motherhood. At what level of labor-market intermittency are women penalized? [special issue]. Am Econ Rev 2003;233–7, 309–14.
[16] Verdon D. Women: half of associates want ownership stake. DVM Newsmagazine 2004;1: 32–5.

[17] Frabotta D. AVPMCA finds burgeoning market in women buyers, joint-practice owners. DVM Newsmagazine 2004;19:47.

[18] Wainer J. Work of female rural doctors. Australian Journal of Rural Health 2004;12(2): 49–53.

[19] Ellsbury KE, Baldwin LM, Johnson KE, et al. Gender-related factors in the recruitment of physicians to the rural Northwest. J Am Board Fam Pract 2002;5:391–400.

[20] Barley GE, Reeves CB, O'Brien-Gonzales A, et al. Characteristics of and issues faced by rural female family physicians. J Rural Health 2001;17(3):251–8.

[21] Pan RJ, Cull WL, Brotherton SE. Pediatric residents' career intentions: data from the leading edge of the pediatrician workforce. Pediatrics 2002;109(2):182–8.

[22] Wise K, editor. Economic report on veterinarians and veterinary practices. Schaumburg (IL): American Veterinary Medical Association 2005.

[23] Volk J, Felsted K, Cummings R, et al. Executive summary of the AVMA-Pfizer business practices study. J Am Vet Med Assoc 2005;226(2):212–8.

[24] American Animal Hospitals Association. Compensation and benefits. 3rd edition. Lakewood (CO): American Animal Hospital Association 2004.

[25] Verdon D. Money worries rank high for most veterinarians. DVM Newsmagazine 2004;19–22.

[26] Major B. From social inequality to personal entitlement: the role of social comparisons, legitimacy appraisals, and group membership. Advances In Experimental Social Psychology 1994;26:293–355.

[27] Major B. Gender differences in comparisons and entitlement: implications for comparable worth. J Soc Issues 1989;45(4):99–115.

[28] Tavris C. Mismeasure of woman: why women are not the better sex, the inferior sex, or the opposite sex. New York: Touchstone Books; 1992.

[29] Feingold A. Cognitive gender differences are disappearing. Am Psychol 1988;43: 95–103.

[30] Rogers L. Sexing the brain. New York: Columbia University Press; 2001. p. 33.

Vet Clin Small Anim 36 (2006) 341–353

VETERINARY CLINICS
SMALL ANIMAL PRACTICE

Current Trends in Animal Law and Their Implications for the Veterinary Profession

Charlotte A. Lacroix, DVM, JD[a,b,*]

[a]Veterinary Business Advisors, Inc., 24 Coddington Road, Whitehouse Station, NJ 08889, USA
[b]University of Pennsylvania School of Veterinary Medicine, Philadelphia, PA, USA

In the last decade the veterinary profession has experienced many changes, which range from the tangible technological advances of renal transplants to the intangible recognition and appreciation of the human–animal bond. Contemporaneous with these changes, the profession and pets have become more visible to the public, and the public has higher expectations for veterinary professional services. The profession also has witnessed the birth of a new area of law, known as "animal law," and an increased scrutiny by the legal community and veterinary state boards.

What do these changes mean to the general practitioner? The veterinary community must keep pace with these changes and in some cases assume a leadership role to protect animals, their owners, and the profession. Veterinarians must participate in and debate the current trends to have an active role in determining how these changes will affect the profession. This article provides a sampling of some of the more challenging issues facing the profession in the early part of the twenty-first century, namely, guardianship versus ownership, the awarding of noneconomic damages in negligence lawsuits, and challenges in maintaining medical records.

GUARDIANSHIP AND NONECONOMIC DAMAGES

For the past several years, pet owners and animal-care industries have been confronted with new legal principles that challenge the way animals have historically been viewed under the law. Although it is no surprise that society's growing compassion for animals and the almost universal embracement of the human–animal bond have led to a greater sensitivity towards the needs of animals and changes in how the law protects animals, this awareness by

*Correspondence. 24 Coddington Road, Whitehouse Station, NJ 08889. E-mail address:
clacroix123@earthlink.net

0195-5616/06/$ – see front matter
doi:10.1016/j.cvsm.2005.10.003

no means justifies a blanket change in the laws that govern the relationship between humans and nonhumans.

Attempts by special-interest groups and animal-law rights advocates to turn the current animal-related laws categorically on their head and apply laws that have formerly applied only to humans without a careful and detailed analysis of the advantages and disadvantages are imprudent. Although most would agree that animals should receive greater protections under current laws and there should be more supervision to ensure animals are treated humanely, the recent proposals to change the status of owners to guardians and award noneconomic damages akin to those awarded for the loss of a human life are excessive measures that create more problems than solutions. Such proposals seem innocuous on their surface but reflect monumental changes in the law.

Two main questions that are currently challenging the veterinary profession, pet owners, and other animal caregivers are whether animal owners should be considered guardians under the law and whether the human–animal bond has monetary value.

Guardianship

Black's Law Dictionary defines property right as "an aggregate of rights which are guaranteed and protected by the government ... the highest right a man can have to anything" [1]. The rights that humans have over nonhumans have been well established for centuries and have reflected society's long-term relationship with animals. As this relationship has evolved, the public has become more sensitive to the needs of animals, and this sensitivity has been reflected in increased legislative activity on animal law issues in both the United States and Europe. Such legislation has attempted, and succeeded in some cases, to impose restrictions on owners' property rights or to remove animals from being treated as property under law.

Although the use of the word "property" offends many, and although it may seem appropriate to use a different term to refer to animals in day-to-day conversation, one must examine whether a change in the terminology as used in legal contexts would be wise in the long run. Some have argued that changing the term "owners" to "guardians" is only a semantic change with no legal significance. Such a statement is disturbing and wrong, because those familiar with legal arguments know full well that there is no such thing as "only semantics" under the law. Lawyers routinely argue before judges about what was or was not meant by simple words. Because guardianship laws are well founded and have universally adopted legal principles, one wonders why a change in terminology would not be interpreted in the same way courts have interpreted its meaning for decades.

Furthermore, while attention is focused on whether the term "guardian" has the same meaning as "owner," the debaters neglect to address whether the "guardian/owner" change in semantics extends to a semantic change between "animal" and "ward." Even if one were to argue that the term "guardian" has the same meaning as the term "owner," no one has stated that the term "ward" has the same meaning as "animal" under current property laws. For example, the change in terminology that was adopted in Rhode Island in 2001 did not address whether a "ward" was created by the adoption of the term "guardian" in lieu of "owner." (The 2001 Cruelty to Animals Law defines guardian as "a person(s) having the same rights and responsibilities of an owner, and both terms shall be used interchangeably. A guardian shall also mean a person who possesses, has title to or an interest in, harbors or has control, custody or possession of an animal and who is responsible for an animal's safety and well-being" [2].) Perhaps this omission was intentional so animal lawyers could establish the point at a later date when representing pets in lawsuits against their "guardians" or other defendants. To say that a parallel semantic change between "animal" and "ward" is implicit and self-evident is unpersuasive.

The laws that govern guardianship are extensive and well established, and it is no coincidence that the term was selected as the substitute for "owner" in current animal-related laws. Under current legal theory, guardians are obligated to care for their "wards" in a manner that subordinates their personal interests. One can only speculate on how this relationship would be applied to animals, but the likely starting point would be the current long-standing definition, that owners have a high duty to exercise care and diligence vis-à-vis their relationship with their animals. Some may argue that guardianship laws would not apply to the owner–animal scenarios because the change is limited to animal anticruelty statutes.

Rhode Island is the only state to have adopted such change in terminology, but many municipalities and cities nationwide have made similar changes, including Wanaque, NJ; Windsor, Ontario, Canada; Berkley, CA; San Francisco, CA; West Hollywood, CA; Boulder, CO; Colorado Springs, CO; Sherwood, AR; Amherst, MA, St. Louis, MO; and Menomonee Falls, WI. Although it is not known how the changes will be interpreted in the future, a complex series of questions invariably come to mind:

- Can guardians treat their own pets?
- Can pets make demands of their guardians?
- Can pets sue their guardians, veterinarians, or the government?
- Can guardians be divested of their property rights?
- Who will pay and provide for care of divested pets?
- Who is responsible for the veterinarian's bill, if care that benefits the pet was not approved by guardian?
- What do shelters do with abandoned animals?
- What if veterinarian disagrees with guardian?

These questions and others are well covered in the white paper authored by a task force of the American Veterinary Medical Law Association, commissioned by the California Veterinary Medical Association and published in 2002 May/June issue of the *California Veterinarian*.

Noneconomic Damages
Closely related to the issue of guardianship is whether the intentional or negligent cause of an animal's death (or injury) should entitle owners to obtain

some form of monetary award to compensate them for their loss. Because veterinarians have been leaders in promoting the human–animal bond, and because they, perhaps better than most, understand the strong relationships owners can have with their pets, it would seem appropriate to allow some form of remedy when a pet has suffered from the wrongful acts of another. Before reacting too quickly in an attempt to do the apparently right thing, however, the profession must carefully examine the current model of noneconomic damages in the human context to determine when such remedies are awarded, when they are not, and why not.

Generally, in the case of human death or injury, courts award both economic and noneconomic damages. Economic damages typically compensate victims for medical bills and the aggregate future income the injured or deceased persons would have earned had they not been harmed. Noneconomic damages, which come in the form of "loss of companionship," "pain and suffering," and "emotional distress damages," can be awarded by courts in cases when the conduct that caused the death or injury was caused by the wrongdoer's intentional act and also in some situations as a result of a tortfeasor's negligent acts, such as medical malpractice.

Courts are inconsistent in awarding noneconomic damages for negligence, in part because negligent acts are based on one's failure to act within the standard of care and typically do not involve intentional misconduct, so awards have little deterrent effect. Noneconomic damages are also awarded only to certain classes of plaintiffs. For example, if an automobile driver's negligence kills a person, none of the person's siblings or best friends are permitted to bring an action for noneconomic damages. Typically, only the deceased person's spouse can sue for such damages. The plaintiffs eligible for such awards vary from state to state, and in some states parents cannot recover noneconomic damages for the death of their child.

Because animals are considered personal property under the law, the amount of monetary damages courts have awarded owners has been based on the fair market value of the animal. This long-standing rule has been applied to the loss of other forms of personal property. This economic remedy historically has been low, unless the animal is a breeding or performance animal. Within the last decade there have been attempts at the legislative and court levels to change the law to allow greater recovery for the loss suffered by those who have lost their animals to the intentional or negligent acts of others.

Only a few states, including, Tennessee and Illinois, have adopted laws that allow a noneconomic remedy for owners who have had animals cruelly injured or killed by violent perpetrators. Additionally, a few states, including Florida, Kentucky, New Jersey, New York, Pennsylvania, and Oregon, allow owners to recover noneconomic damages for the "intentional infliction of emotional distress" that the owners can prove they suffered from the death or injury of an animal as a result of a wrongdoer's reckless, extreme, and outrageous misconduct. Except for Tennessee, the author is unaware of any laws that permit noneconomic damages as a remedy for negligent acts, and most courts that have addressed the issue of whether noneconomic damages are appropriate for actions caused by negligence when there is no cruelty, recklessness, or intentional misconduct have concluded that such a remedy is inappropriate and not in the best interest of the public.

For example, in a September 2004 court decision that was based on a veterinary malpractice case in which the veterinarian had been found negligent for having failed to diagnose a gastrointestinal obstruction in a timely manner, the Superior Court of New Jersey concluded that based on "public policy reasons, non-economic damages for the negligent death of a pet should not be recognized as a matter of law" [3]. In arriving at its opinion, the Superior Court's decision referenced a Wisconsin court's concerns [4]:

> [W]ere such a claim to go forward, the law would proceed upon a course that had no just stopping point. Humans have an enormous capacity to form bonds with dogs, cats, birds and an infinite number of other beings that are non-human. Were we to recognize a claim for damages for the negligent loss of a dog, we can find little basis for rationally distinguishing other categories of animal companion. ... [T]he public policy concerns relating to identifying genuine claims of emotional distress, as well as charging tortfeasors with financial burdens that are fair, compel the conclusion [not to award such damages].

The correctness of the decision by most courts not to award noneconomic damages for the negligent loss or injury of an animal is currently being debated. Given that the current laws allow such awards for loss of human lives, but such awards are not available for the loss of a person's sibling, best friend, or same-sex partner, it would be inequitable and troublesome to allow such a remedy for the loss of an animal.

Conclusion

The issues of whether pets should be treated as "children" under the law and whether noneconomic damages should be awarded for negligent acts are challenging veterinarians' ability to conduct their practices as usual and the ethical paradigm to which they have grown accustomed. It is important to recognize that social change is occurring, but it is even more important to avoid reacting too quickly and making the wrong decision because of incorrect assumptions about the social change.

MEDICAL RECORDS: A FACT OF GOOD AND DEFENSIBLE PRACTICE

Of all the changes the profession will need to embrace within the next few years, maintaining proper and complete medical records is by far the most important. Veterinary medicine has advanced to extend the lives of and provide a better quality of life for animals and their owners through high-quality preventative and medical health care. Unfortunately, veterinary record-keeping has not evolved in a similar fashion. Over a 20-year period (1985–2005), 414 disciplinary actions were taken by the Texas Board of Veterinary Medical Examiners.

Record-keeping issues, including failure to maintain Drug Enforcement Agency (DEA) logs, were involved in 32% of those actions, followed by standard-of-care violations (30%) and license/continuing education violations (27%) [5]. Texas is not alone on this issue. The Florida Board of Veterinary Medicine issued 51 disciplinary actions between October 2001 and October 2003; of those, 27 (53%) involved a failure to maintain proper records [6].

Why is it that, within 6 months of graduation, most veterinary school graduates fail to maintain their medical records properly, a skill they were required to master in their fourth year? The most popular excuses include "I don't have time," "my boss doesn't do it," and "I no longer need to demonstrate my competence to a faculty member." What most new graduates and their more senior colleagues must understand is that proper medical record keeping is directly correlated with the quality of medicine delivered and is inversely correlated with the number of malpractice lawsuits won by plaintiffs. With more than 40 law schools teaching animal law and veterinary malpractice to their law students, and with the increased number of complaints filed with veterinary state boards nationwide, it behooves prudent veterinarians to re-examine their record-keeping practices. Veterinarians can no longer afford to be insensitive to the details of maintaining proper medical records.

Importance of Medical Records

The key to understanding what and how much information should be in a medical record lies in understanding the fundamental purposes of the medical record, which are twofold. The medical record is an evidentiary document generated to communicate to others what was done and why it was done or, if not done, why it was not done. The information within medical records must explain and substantiate a veterinarian's actions or omissions. The Pennsylvania Practice Act under §31.22 [7] states this purpose clearly:

> Veterinary medical records serve as a basis for planning animal care and as a means of communication among members of the veterinary practice. The records furnish documentary evidence of the animal's illness, hospital care and treatment and serve as a basis for review, study and evaluation of the care and treatment rendered by the veterinarian.

The shortcomings of most medical records are that they do not contain sufficient information to access the veterinarian's actions or inactions and do not present the information so that the reader can follow the cognitive reasoning of the veterinarian. Too frequently, furthermore, the information is illegible. Although veterinarians are not expected to give a dissertation on the medical treatment of a patient, they should document defensively, as if they expected to be questioned later about their decisions and actions.

The second fundamental purpose of medical records is that they are necessary to provide ongoing quality medical care. Because entries in medical records should be recorded contemporaneously with the events they record, the medical record serves as a chronologic medical map of a patient's diagnoses and treatments. From this map, the treating veterinarian can more easily generate a mental algorithm that reflects a logical medical rationale, thereby increasing the likelihood of successful treatment. One of the main complaints of specialists and emergency clinicians is that they are unable to pick up where the referring veterinarian left off because the poor quality (or in some instances, nonexistence) of records makes it impossible to follow a logical medical rationale. Referral and emergency hospitals are becoming more widely used, and good records are essential aids in the appropriate assessment, diagnosis, and treatment of referred patients.

Medical Record Information

Medical records typically encompass the patient records of individual pets but also include the business and legal documents of the hospital, such as estimates, invoices, hospital handouts, financial records, and all logs. In acts or regulations many states set the minimum information that must be included in medical records. Other good resources include the American Animal Hospital Association (AAHA) guidelines for an accredited hospitals on the AAHA Website [8] and current articles in publications such as *Veterinary Economics* [9].

Generally, the amount and type of information recorded should be consistent with the level and complexity of the services rendered. The most common information veterinarians fail to include in the medical record is communications with the client, staff, and colleagues regarding the care of the patient. This omission probably occurs because, when the communication takes place, the medical record is nowhere to be found; most practices are not sufficiently organized to make locating the record any easier than finding a needle in a haystack. Fortunately, advances in computer and intercom technology are helping reduce this administrative nightmare. Certain information should not be recorded: under no circumstances should medical records include derogatory statements about clients, patients, or colleagues, because such comments invariably come back and crush the credibility of the author.

The information and documents that constitute medical records include

A. Medical (Initial all entries and corrections.)
  1. Client admission forms: client (name, address, contact information); patient ID (name, species, age, sex); emergency contact person and contact information
  2. Client consents: recommendations, requests contrary to recommendations, refusals/acceptance of recommendations
    a. Euthanasia
    b. High-risk surgeries (or any surgery)
    c. Sterilizations
    d. Legal cosmetic procedures
    e. Necropsies
    f. Hospitalizations
  3. Medical history and treatment chart
    a. Date and time of hospital visit

      b. Vaccination and medical history, chief complaint
      c. Physical examination: abnormal, normal, or not examined; weight
      d. Diagnosis: master problem list with diagnosis and with prognosis if applicable
      e. Treatment: medical and surgical; state medications (dosages in mg, not mL) (Include all options, let clients make treatment decisions and have sign off on them.)
      f. Final assessment of patient
      g. Home-care instructions to clients
    4. Radiographs, laboratory data, surgical and dental reports
    5. Client education: preventative health care list/professional advice rendered
    6. Client communications/correspondence
    7. Colleague communications
    8. Large animals
      a. Conversation logs with date, time, and summary of discussion
      b. Dates and dosages of all medications administered to animals, including route of administration and concentration of dosages, withdrawal periods
      c. Instructions left with clients
      d. Feed additives prescribed with dosages and withdrawal periods
      e. Documentation that the client understands the requisite withdrawal periods
      f. Procedures used to prevent transfer of zoonotic disease from one farm to another
      g. ID of all treated animals (encourage producers to place permanent ID.)
      h. Recommendations to clients of potential contamination risks; observations and conversations
  B. Business/legal
    1. Estimates and invoices
    2. Appointment books
    3. Hospital handouts
    4. Financial records
    5. Surgery, radiograph, laboratory, and DEA logs
      a. Surgery log
        (1) Animal's and owner's names
        (2) Surgeon's name
        (3) Type of surgical procedure
        (4) Length of time of surgery
        (5) Type and amount of preanesthetic and anesthetic agents
        (6) Complications/problems
        (7) Any other pertinent information related to patient (health status) or procedure (surgical support team)
      b. Radiology log
        (1) Date
        (2) Type of study (eg, abdomen)
        (3) Animal's and owner's names
        (4) Technician's name

(5) Exposure factors
(6) Reference number
c. DEA/narcotic log
(1) Inventory of drugs
(2) Date purchased and amts
(3) Usage of drugs, including who, amount, when

The information maintained in the medical records is much more useful if it is kept current. As do medical practitioners treating humans, veterinarians should have their clients update admission information annually. Too often circumstances arise that require veterinarians and their staff to determine who has the authority to make decisions pertaining to a patient's medical care, and information as basic as who owns the pet is lacking. For example, in a world in which divorced couples fight for custody rights of their pets and owners claim that euthanasia was not properly authorized, veterinarians must be extremely diligent and meticulous in obtaining correct and complete information on their patients.

Confidentiality of Medical Records

Protecting personal information of clients is an ethical duty for all veterinarians and is a legal duty in about 22 states (Table 1). The 2002 revision of the American Veterinary Medical Association Principles of Veterinary Medical Ethics under Principle II (L) states

> Veterinarians and their associates should protect the personal privacy of patients and clients. Veterinarians should not reveal confidences unless required to by law or unless it becomes necessary to protect the health and welfare of other individuals or animals.

Even in states that do not have explicit prohibitions on divulging confidential client information, veterinarians should exercise caution before revealing client information to a third party. Always attempt to obtain the client's consent and, in cases of emergency such as when the health of a person or pet is at risk, be sure there is a paper trail that justifies the disclosure of the confidential information.

Challenges of the Paperless Practice

The paperless office is a popular trend in veterinary practice management but is not suitable for everyone. Those who think that a paperless practice is the answer to their woes should remember that bad record keeping can only be magnified through electronics. Computer systems can be laborious and time consuming if not used properly. Practitioners who are thinking about transitioning to a paperless practice should consider (1) doing a cost-benefit analysis, (2) whether the staff and doctors have the organizational skills and acumen to implement the standardized operating procedures necessary for a paperless

Table 1
States requiring confidentiality of client information

State	Citation	Summary of cited references
Alabama	930-X-1-.11 (15)	A veterinarian shall not violate the confidential relationship between himself or herself and his or her client.
Alaska	12 AAC 68.910 (d)	Patient medical records may not be released to a third party without written consent of the owner.
California	Bus. and Prof. Code § 4857; Civ. Proc. § 1985.3	Veterinarian shall not disclose information related to the client, the animal, or the services rendered except with written or electronic authorization from the client, a court order/subpoena, or has required to comply with laws. Proceedings/records of organized committee meetings of vet hospital staff not subject to discovery.
Delaware	24 oe 3313 (1)	Prohibits willful violation of any privileged communication
Georgia	24-9-29 50-18-17 (a)	No veterinarian shall be required to disclose any information concerning the veterinarian's care of any animal except on written authorization or other waiver by the veterinarian's client of an appropriate court order or subpoena. Medical or veterinary or similar files, the disclosure of which would be an invasion of privacy, are considered confidential.
Idaho	IDAPA 46-013	Incorporates by reference the AVMA Principles of Veterinary Medical Ethics
Illinois	225 ILLCS 115/25/17	No veterinarian shall be required to disclose any information concerning the veterinarian's care of any animal except on written authorization or other waiver by the veterinarian's client or an appropriate court order or subpoena When communicable disease laws, cruelty to animals laws, or laws providing for public health or safety are involved, this privilege is waived.
Kansas	47-839	No veterinarian ... shall be required to disclose any information concerning the veterinarian's care of a n animal, except on written authorization or other waiver by the veterinarian's client or an appropriate court order or subpoena.

Table 1
(*continued*)

State	Citation	Summary of cited references
Kentucky	201 KAR 16:010 Sec. 23	A veterinarian shall maintain a confidential relationship with his client, except as otherwise provided by law, or required by considerations related to public health or animal health
Massachusetts	256 CMR: 7.01 (15)	A veterinarian shall maintain a confidential relationship with his/her clients, except as otherwise provided by law or required by considerations related to public health and/or animal health.
Minnesota	156.081 2 (14)	Prohibits revealing a privileged communication from or relating to a client except when otherwise required or permitted by law
Missouri	4-270-6.011 (11)	Licensees shall not reveal confidential, proprietary, or privileged facts or data or any other sensitive information contained in a patient's medical records or as otherwise obtained in a professional capacity without prior consent of the client except as required by the board, court order, or law or regulation.
Montana	37-1-316 (9)	Revealing confidential information obtained as a result of a professional relationship without the prior consent of the recipient of services, except as authorized or required by law constitutes unprofessional conduct.
New Hampshire	501.01	Incorporates by reference the AVMA Principles of Veterinary Medical Ethics
Nebraska	71-148 (9)	Willfully betraying a professional secret except as otherwise provided by law constitutes unprofessional conduct.
Oklahoma	10-5-15	A licensed veterinarian shall not violate the confidential relations between himself and his client.
Pennsylvania	49 OE 31.21 Principle 7 (c)	Veterinarians and their staff shall protect the personal privacy of clients, unless the veterinarians are required by law to reveal the confidences or it becomes necessary to reveal the confidences to protect the health and welfare of an individual, the animal, or others whose health and welfare may be endangered.

Table 1
(continued)

State	Citation	Summary of cited references
Tennessee	1730-1.13 (6)	It is unprofessional conduct to reveal without written permission knowledge obtained in a professional capacity about animals or owners. Exceptions (b) are to other law enforcement agencies.
Texas	4-801.353	Veterinarian may not violate the confidential relationship between the veterinarian and the veterinarian's client. Veterinarian may not be required to release information unless written consent of or waiver by client or subpoena/court order or the board
Virginia	150-20-140.4 150-20-170	Unprofessional conduct shall include violating the confidential relationship between a veterinarian and his client. Unprofessional conduct includes compromising the confidentiality of the doctor/client relationship.
West Virginia	26-4-2.14	A licensed veterinarian shall not violate his or her confidential relationship with the client.
Wyoming	Chp 4 Sec 1(b) Chp 4 Sec 3 d vi	Incorporates by reference the AVMA Principles of Veterinary Medical Ethics Contents of medical records shall be kept confidential and not released to third parties unless authorized by the client or required by law.

Abbreviation: AVMA, American Veterinary Medical Association.

Data from As revised by Gregory M. Dennis, Esq., of Kent T. Perry & Co., L.C., Overland Park, Kansas; American Society for the Prevention of Cruelty to Animals; and Gary J. Patronek, VMD, PhD, Tufts University School of Veterinary Medicine, Grafton, MA.

system to work, (3) whether the practices should use wireless technology and the use of desktop computers versus laptops or personal digital assistants, and, most importantly, (4) whether the staff is ready to implement and embrace the change. The attitude of the staff is often more challenging than the technological challenges.

The laws and requirements regarding electronic records generally include the necessity for an audit trail (chain of custody) with the record being unalterable after a certain period of time (eg, 24 hours), the purpose being to allow limited access to changing the files by necessitating new entries for corrections and having all updates or deletions automatically noted on the record. Authentication through password protection, voiceprints, and user-identification technology is also essential. Finally, the ability to back up the files reliably is critical, especially if records are requested by the veterinary state board of examiners or local plaintiff's attorney. It is a good idea to contact the veterinary state board to determine if the practice act or its regulations have any guidelines or requirements that should be met by paperless practices.

SUMMARY

Relative to other professionals, veterinarians as a whole have had few complaints to the state board and negligence lawsuits filed against them. This situation has led to an industry-wide problem of complacency concerning medical record-keeping practices. Fortunately, most veterinarians spend their days being challenged by medicine and adopting preventative medical procedures rather than being preoccupied with managing risks associated with malpractice lawsuits. Unfortunately, with the rising interest in issues related to animal law, the veterinary professionals will need to adopt practices that ensure that medical records are complete, accurate, and easily accessible.

References

[1] Nolan JR, Nolan-Haley JM. Black's law dictionary. 6th edition. St. Paul (MN): West Publishing Co.; 1990. p. 1216.
[2] Rhode Island, Animals and Animal Husbandry, Title 4, Section 4-1-1 (2005).
[3] *Frampton v. Allenwood Animal Hospital*, (Docket No. A-2154–03T3).
[4] *Rideau v. City of Racine*, 243 Wis.2d 486, 627 N.W.2d 795, 798–802 (2001).
[5] Texas State Board of Veterinary Medical Examiners. Disciplinary Actions (A-L & M-Z). Available at: http://www.tbvme.state.tx.us/disciplinary.htm. Accessed May 2005.
[6] Florida Department of Business and Professional Regulation, Board of Veterinary Medicine. Disciplinary Cases. Newsletter 2004;(Spring):4–7.
[7] Pennsylvania State Board of Veterinary Medicine Regulations 49§31.22.
[8] American Animal Hospital Association Standards of Accreditation (2003 revision). Available at: http://www.aahanet.org/Stand/Index.html. Accessed May 2005.
[9] Guenther J. Industry issues, part 2: 10 key rules for record keeping. Veterinary Economics 2004;45:62–5.

Vet Clin Small Anim 36 (2006) 355–371

VETERINARY CLINICS
SMALL ANIMAL PRACTICE

Succession Planning

Thomas E. Catanzaro, DVM, MHA

Veterinary Practice Consultants, 18301 W. Colfax Avenue (R-101), Golden, CO 80401, USA

"All business proceeds on beliefs, or judgements, or probabilities, and not on certainties."—Charles W. Eliot

Succession planning is the slow but deliberate process of altering the leadership structure of the practice to better prepare for tomorrow. The succession planning experienced by most practice owners wishing to sell in the new millennium is not what they encountered when they entered practice 30 to 50 years ago. The sellers are predominantly Baby Boomers (born in 1946 to 1967), with a few of the Silent Majority (born before 1946). Most existing practice owners entered into a sparse veterinary density market or developed a companion animal practice from an ambulatory heritage practice. The buyers are mostly Generation X (born in 1968 to 1990) veterinarians, with a few transient Baby Boomers, entering a dense veterinary density market (except for mixed animal practices, which are finding it almost impossible to find new associates, much less buyers). These generational groups not only expect different things from their profession but also have different vocabularies and different basic professional values.

One of the most significant challenges facing the veterinary profession is not competition or recession but the ability to change the habits that got us where we are today. This fact is behind the adage, "If you are satisfied with what you've done to get where you are, you will stagnate and die." The influx of corporate America into the veterinary profession reflects two emerging parameters: (1) there is money to be made, and (2) the traditional veterinary health care delivery systems (isolationism) of the 1970s and 1980s are not serving the needs of the community. Tucker in his book entitled *Managing the Future* [1] has captured many of these concepts and categorized ten driving forces of change as we enter the new millennium, specifically, factors that influence the consumer's behavior. I have used Tucker's ten forces and my consulting experience to apply these driving forces to situations that most practices encounter today.

E-mail address: drtomcat@aol.com

0195-5616/06/$ – see front matter
doi:10.1016/j.cvsm.2005.11.004

DYNAMICS OF CHANGE

Tucker makes a great opening statement that needs to be remembered, "The best way to predict the future is to invent it!" The leadership text *Building the Successful Veterinary Practice: Innovation & Creativity* [2] explores the learning organization and the creative process that leaders can instill. The premise of change management is that one first needs to create some form of dissatisfaction or discomfort centered on a specific habit (eg, vaccine price sensitivity owing to large format retailer "media blitz" efforts) and not with life or the practice. Second, one needs to find an alternative model, that is, something that anticipates future needs (eg, 10-minute, fast-in fast-out, nurse-based, wellness vaccination appointments). The third step is to develop the process of change or the constant reinforcement of the new model in operation until it becomes habit (eg, preferred client access to these "economic benefit" programs). In more simple terms, the process is as follows:

> Unfreeze the old habit.
> Reform the specific activity into a new shape or model.
> Refreeze the new model into a habit.

If we look at superstores offering pet health care, veterinary public-owned complexes, or affiliated practice markets, economies of scale help them to some degree; however, the real reason for their success is that they see veterinary medicine as a business and make business decisions on a regular basis. They are not going to go away, nor can an individual practitioner effectively compete with them on their playing field. The secret to practice success is defining one's own playing field, and the key to succession planning is to have a clear 3- to 10-year plan of practice transition for the new ownership to assume practice leadership. Revolutionary (not evolutionary) success lies in making business decisions in one's own practice while not worrying about the other practice. There are three main reasons for this practice owner attitude:

> As long as you blame someone or something else, you will never decide to cope with the realization that you must control your own environment. You must change and adapt to the changing community.
> Positive thought begets positive action, whereas negative thought begets negative action. Health care must be a positive environment to succeed.
> Every practice has areas where services may be enhanced, especially in wellness surveillance, an emerging profession initiative (http://www.npwm.com), where programs may be expanded, or even areas where some process continues because "it's always been that way," a sure sign of a need to change!

SUCCESSION PLANNING

The only thing certain about tomorrow is that you cannot stop it from coming. Thirty years ago, veterinary medicine averaged one doctor per practice, and it took a population of about 10,000 to support a full-time veterinarian. Today, practices have an average of 2.5 doctors and a population of 4000 clients per full-time equivalent veterinarian. Thirty years ago, the one-doctor practice had a value between $250,000 and $300,000. Today, the 2.5-doctor practice has an estimated value in the $900,000 plus range. At 20% down, the one-doctor practice was within the reach of most practitioners for purchase, whereas few professional individuals can raise the $150,000 plus down payment needed to procure a veterinary practice today. There is a much greater need for practice owners to develop a succession plan for ownership, and the author and his colleagues are called in more often to help with the transition.

SUCCESSION EXAMPLES

Dr. A.L. was the patriarch of his practice, supported quietly by his wife (she was a wonderful practice asset). He hired an associate and put her on a developmental program, and eventually she used her "minority status" to buy half of the practice with government money. The practice grew to 3.5 doctors (the patriarch was the half-time practitioner). He had cardiac bypass surgery and needed the associate to assume more accountability for the practice, but she was not ready and resisted. He reassumed the role of patriarch, and a status quo emerged until the health of his wife and his own energy forced the succession issue to re-emerge. We had to build a system of support from within the staff to support the new owner, but she was not the decisive owner envisioned by the patriarch. He still fights to become comfortable enough with her style to let go of the practice operations.

Dr. P.R. had retired in place but still operated his practice as a small one-doctor practice. There had been no growth; the annual gross had been $175,000 ± $25,000 for the past 4 years; and the facility was not current. He wanted to sell, but no one was interested in an outdated practice with one examination room and no surgical facility. We started with the facility and proposed an inpatient expansion, constructed at only 12% of what a "veterinary-specific architect" estimated an expansion would cost. We added an entry level, single-station, veterinary computer system and upgraded the patient advocacy of the doctor. Within 4 months, he reached the point where $1000 days were the minimum, and he was routinely cresting to $2000 plus days during the busy seasons. He began having fun and experiencing pride again and decided not to retire immediately. After 3 years, we were ready to market the practice but had to start from scratch because the associate we had added and developed over 2 years decided in the eleventh hour that she did not want to commit to the practice purchase.

Drs. R & A had a mixed animal practice, were married (to each other), and needed relief; therefore, they brought another couple into the practice as associates. The relationship was solid and eventually Drs. R & A sold a share of the practice to them. Two couples (four doctors) were owners of a solid three-doctor practice. As such, they had to hire an unneeded associate to allow the couples to each take appropriate time off. The partnership agreement also called for a sabbatical arrangement; however, to take off long periods, the business operations had to be transferred slowly to the new ownership couple, something the new ownership pair did not really desire. We had to build a system of operational management tracking that the new couple could monitor and manage while giving them a better cash flow to allow the hiring of an additional associate during the sabbatical (actually hired by the couple on sabbatical from their partnership monies).

Over his career, Dr. G.B. had built a successful three-facility complex, had established his retirement plan early, and had invested wisely in stocks, real estate, and other assets. His son had joined the practice; there were three other associates with over a decade of tenure each; and Dr. G.B. had a good handle on the programs and procedures that caused liquidity. When he was ready to retire, he simply gave the four doctors (son plus three) 24% of the practice each with the simple explanation that he had all the money he wanted, three homes, and had already educated his family. Problems occurred when the four doctors could not replicate what the one doctor had done. Their attempt at management was "number heavy" (comparing percentages) but without common sense or a program/procedure basis. We had to recalibrate the team and their approach and help them realize that each of the three practices were different entities. We also had to reintroduce the "program-based" budget system, which was common to the original owner's technique of leadership (he did not call it program-based budgeting, but his logic was client centered and procedure smart).

RULES OF THUMB
As a rule of thumb, I hate rules of thumb. Regardless, some guidelines are needed to start the discussions herein. Some of these rules are common sense; therefore, the reader is asked to take each with a "grain of NaCl."

- The banks, small business administration, and other lenders will not lend money on blue sky (eg, goodwill, projected earnings); therefore, a down payment is needed in most practice sale deals unless you are willing to carry the paper.
- The building and land should be in a separate "land and cattle company" (LLC, family trust, or some other shelter), and you should be paying yourself a reasonable rent (eg, 7% to 10%). This setup saves federal taxes every month, as well as at the end of your career, especially if the real estate entity in not within the practice owner's estate.
- If the practice is solely owned and there are multiple associates, consider developing a stock-based ownership structure so that a junior partner within your tenured professional team can elect a "stair-step" purchase option, which allows small percentages of shares to be purchased systematically by the favored doctor over a prolonged period.
- If the practice has many partners and few associates, ensure that you have some form of "first death" protection insurance. The ownership of the policy needs to belong to a legal entity other than yourself (to keep the proceeds out of the ever-changing estate tax), and the beneficiary needs to be kept current (again, it should not be the practice entity for estate and taxation reasons).
- The old valuation system of taking 70% to 80% of the annualized average of 3 years' gross as the practice price is valid only if (1) there has been 15% to 20% net growth annually; (2) there is no debt; and (3) someone is willing to

buy it at that price (it is rare to find this point combination in the current buyer's market). The Association of Veterinary Practice Management Consultants and Advisors (AVPMCA) Task Force spent over 2 years developing 12 AVPMCA risk factors (http://www.avpmca.org). These factors are becoming the preferred and more accurate factors for establishing the capitalization rate and the real value of the average companion animal practice. Accountant valuations that use earnings before interest, taxes, depreciation, and amortization (EBITDA) multiples or that do not address the AVPMCA's 12 risk factors can no longer be trusted to be acceptable in the buyer's market place. Specialty practices and food animal practices usually have a value in real assets but little else because they are personal relationship–based practices. Reputations can carry such practices to some form of partnership or shared ownership for an established associate, and these transitions are essential to increase the practice value for the new buyer or the seller at retirement.

- The practice sale preparation needs to start at least 3 years before the anticipated separation date because net must be increased (every valuation formula is "net sensitive"). Actually, 5 years before the anticipated sale, smart sellers quit laundering money through the practice (hiding expenses and salaries). In the fourth year, the sellers establish a growth and promotion plan that will cause a growing practice profile over the next half decade.
- The transition of ownership and practice leadership must be initiated a full business cycle before the anticipated retirement date because the practice's leadership must be transferred smoothly for the purpose of staff and client retention. This transition often requires a mediator (a qualified consultant and mentor) to assist all parties in maintaining harmony and practice pride. Quality is what the client calls pride.
- If you are a young practitioner, start banking or investing 10% of your take-home pay every month effective immediately with no excuses. Also, at the end of every year, whether you are a practice owner or a productivity-based associate getting an end-of-year bonus, place 50% of the excess net bonus into solid real estate land investments in your community. In this manner, the practice sale becomes supplemental money and not primary retirement money.

These points are made simply because too many practices fail to plan ahead, and because the public veterinary corporations are not always the answer. If you cannot see your practice days ending or you only see one method of exit, succession planning is even more critical. Succession planning is how to move from one level of your veterinary medical evolution to the next level of your life. It needs to be done today and committed to completely, regardless of the evolutionary level you are at, because life and family are long lasting, whereas practice is transitory. Today is already yesterday's tomorrow, and nothing stopped it from happening. Learn from that fact, plan for the future, and it will not be scary.

WHAT IS YOUR PRACTICE WORTH?

The usual way of looking at practice value is to estimate the sum of the money an owner might get by selling the practice. This amount is best expressed as a sum of the assets and the return over expenses, although, in reality, it is only what someone is willing to pay for the practice. Contrary to certified public accountant versions of valuation, the assets of the practice are much greater than the monetary price. The only thing all of the assets have in common is that they need to undergo regular maintenance by people and to be in a constant state of improvement, involving an in-depth, skill-based discussion of continuous quality improvement by well-led teams.

We all recognize that beyond the cash and equipment in a practice value, there are human assets. Beyond the human assets are the visions of the owners, leaders, and staff. The discussion of value becomes wider than just bookkeeping. Vision is more than expense control. Succession planning is sharing the plan and not just selling.

"It's what you do with what you got that counts."—Lesley Dunlap

One of the most underused practice assets is the staff. Maintaining their value means enlisting their brains and hearts as well as their bodies for practice enhancement. Staff members need to know why something is happening, especially if they are the ones who are supposed to tell the clients why something is important. The staff is the first market for any program; if they are not "sold" on the concept, there will be no pride. If there is no pride, the effort will never succeed. In succession planning, this means the following:

- It is becoming far smarter to "grow your own" successor than trying to sell the practice on the open market.
- One should invest outside the practice, build independent retirement resources by small investments each month, and legally separate the building/land from the practice so that "landlord money" can continue after the practice stops.
- It is essential to start "letting go" of the control that built your success when the practice approaches a two-doctor setup.
- Delegation to others requires training to a level of trust, persuasion of others that they can do it, and coaching to fine-tune skills and knowledge.

Paraprofessional and professional staff, as well as owners, need to be nurtured. Respect, responsibility, and recognition are the key three elements in an organization's environment. If we assume that these three elements exist in the practice environment, we must address another critical element of the top six staff satisfaction elements—a quality compensation program. This element is seldom in the top three motivators of belonging, responsibility, and contribution/self-esteem but is always in the top six expectations. If one expects to "grow succession elements" from within, there must be a livable wage (with benefits) and a retirement plan that makes people want to stay.

There are many ways that money appears as the "root of all evil," but without it, nothing else can occur. In fact, without it, the front door is locked by the bank and can never swing again. The major problem in veterinary medicine is that it is a young profession in which business is defined as we go. The first companion animal hospital was built in 1929, and the American Animal Hospital Association was started in 1938. Almost all practice owners learned from a male veterinarian (the sex of virtually all practitioners at that time) who was in a farm practice and who decided to see the "smaller critters," the reason why we call it "small animal medicine." A review of the following habits and traditions, and the alternatives, provides insight (Box 1)

Money does matter, and it must be captured from the work we do. Veterinary medicine is a fee-for-service business; products are only supportive; and, in companion animal practice, we generally treat patients that are considered "family members" (as shown in the original family value research published in *The Pet Connection*) [5]. We deal in needs of the patient, the client, and the provider (which includes all staff members of a practice). Most of these factors are discussed in detail in the text, *Beyond the Successful Veterinary Practice: Succession Planning & Other Legal Issues* [6].

ANNUAL PROGRAM-BASED BUDGET

> "Budgeting is often a daunting activity, approached in some companies with a strange mixture of disinterest and awe."—Robert G. Finney

The program-based budget lies at the absolute epicenter of practice activities, not as the driver, the dictator, or the demon, but the mile marker to success. It is similar to the famous Rod of the Old Testament Proverbs. Actually, in today's dynamic marketplace, it is more like the scorecard of golf or the tote board at the racetrack. It is a fiscal-based scorecard that gives the odds and handicapped assessment of success with programs and procedures. It exists not to beat down staff members but to serve as a standard of excellence when looking at the commitments made by the practice providers to the standards of care of the practice. A program-based budget will provide targets and measurement for your vision and outcome expectations; however, you must discuss the science of the procedures, what clients need to hear, and what patients deserve. Money is the silent outcome of consistently solid program delivery. Although not every activity needs to make a "pure mega-profit," the decision has to be yours. Losses, on the other hand, should be avoided. When the veterinary chart of accounts is married to the practice operations, you will begin to see the practice value you need to maintain.

Line item accounting has always been done by traditional accountants for expenses, whereas they have ignored line items for income centers. This approach is called "dumb accounting" by everyone except the accountant sending you the bill. These are the same people who seldom spell accounting with an "A." Their fees are often hidden from you under the categories of "legal" or "professional" because they alphabetize the profit and loss for their own benefit, not yours, and do not want to be at the top of the list. Even with food sales, one of the smallest mark-up activities in a practice, break-even analysis means you must know what is being spent and compare that with what is being sold in real dollars. To know what is being sold, the beginning and ending inventory must be computed with the purchases to identify the real value of what was sold. This amount is compared with the nutritional product sales. With maintenance diets, a 20% to 25% net is expected;

Box 1: Veterinary practice habits, traditions, alternatives

− We have routinely scheduled one doctor in one consult room with a single column of clients, yet physicians use four to six rooms per doctor, and dentists are able to double that number (think of the old-time veterinarian in their truck doing one farm at a time).

+ If you believe in the new American veterinary practice and understand that "staff produces the net," review high-density scheduling concepts for some alternative methods (http://www.v-p-c.com).

− We have routinely charged anesthesia based on the animal size, yet isoflurane only costs about $6 per hour to use (think of the value of the cow in the chute, the veterinarian and his black bag, and the cost per pound to make her well).

+ If you want the new American veterinary practice, consider the following sequence with each item/procedure deserving its own fair price:

  Preanesthetic blood screen (varies with age and physical condition)

  Presurgery pain management [3]

  Intravenous (to keep open) slow fluid drip

  Induction (less than $20, but covers most overhead)

  Initial maintenance (not by weight, but for 30 minutes minimum)

  Continuing anesthesia maintenance (by the minute)

  Postsurgery pain management

  Episodal hospitalization

  Follow-up plan

− The old-timers made preanesthesia blood screening voluntary, intravenous supportive therapy during surgery an exception, and always said, "but what about the price?"

+ In quality practices, the blood screen is now mandatory (is minimum and preferred, two yes options).

+ In progressive practices that worry about animal pain and rapid recovery, supportive intravenous therapy during surgery is mandatory.

+ Postsurgical pain management is an expectation of most clients and forgotten by the provider owing to "wallet medicine."

+ Pricing is secondary to the need of the patient and the need of the provider in quality care. Compromise of professional standards is a liability.

− We have always charged hospitalization cage and run space by the animal size (almost like a feedlot operation).

+ The value is in the time, process, and people involved, not in the kibble in the bowl:

  Day admit cases—level one hospitalization

  Once daily/twice daily cases—level two hospitalization

  Three times a day/four times a day cases—level three hospitalization

  Intravenous cases—level four hospitalization (also post surgery)

  Intensive care unit cases—level five hospitalization

+ This method of value measurement can also be used in bandaging (no joint, one joint, two joint, with an appliance or supportive wrap or without). Start re-thinking your habits!

− We have always been afraid to sell our knowledge and instead have routinely sold "things" (eg, vaccines at major inflation mark-ups, the cost of the examination instead of the doctor's consultation).

+ Production veterinarians have started charging for their time, even on the telephone, with clients.

+ Production veterinarians have started software computer systems to manage husbandry for their clients and charge for this service.

+ Production and ambulatory veterinarians charge by the mile to get to a client, yet specialists who travel between companion animal practices usually do not.

+ When the pendulum swings, why do the companion animal veterinarians always wait for the "other guys" to change first?

− We have always managed companion animal practices by expense comparisons, yet traditional veterinary software has been developed much like fancy cash registers, tracking only income factors (and a mail merge for client mailings).

+ Without expense-to-income relationships, you cannot determine net.

+ Program-based budgeting [4] provides program and procedure factors for managing practices—the things that make the front door swing!

+ The new emerging veterinary software systems, with 32-bit Windows technology, track health care delivery from the medical records instead of the invoice, in picture and word, and the better systems also have automatic data download capabilities to problem lists as well as existing spreadsheet programs for easy practice use.

+, good insight; −, bad paradigm.

with a heavy prescription diet program, a 35% to 40% net is expected. Break-even analysis means ensuring the internal controls are adequate to maintain these levels of net. This level of managerial accounting is needed for the best resale of a practice, although it is not needed for Internal Revenue Service (IRS) tax accounting.

The budget-to-actual computations made each month are a combination of internal controls, break-even analysis, and quality assurance. The cost-per-use of a new piece of equipment is a form of break-even analysis, but a practice may not always be able to charge that much. The health care delivery team may use the cost-per-use as a method to establish a target of how many uses the practice must perform each month to break even (eg, Cardell blood pressure monitoring in consultation rooms, along with a Biolog lead II rhythm strip, dry chemistry and electrolyte machines, Vetronics ECG, endoscope, ultrasound machine, new dental base). Once the equipment-specific break-even point is determined and the number of procedures computed to carry the cost, every procedure past this number is pure profit.

THE URGE TO MERGE

"There are risks and costs to a program of action, but they are far less than the long-range risks and costs of comfortable inaction."—John F. Kennedy

As a consultant, what I have done in all mergers is become the "champion of the outcome." This support model has proven most successful for human health care consultants. I have encountered veterinary consultants who fight for their client as if a merger was a win-lose negotiation. This approach causes failure to be built into the negotiations (Box 2). As a result, this section is written from the champion of the outcome perspective.

The first critical question to be addressed is why merge or why affiliate. What is the rationale for the concept? There are four factors: market, cost, community, and system. The market is geography based in veterinary medicine, with the impact on the share of market enjoyed. The cost addresses economies of scale and expense avoidance factors. The community is the benefactor of the consolidation and collaboration, when a quality and continuity of care ensues. The system of health care delivery becomes integrated, management develops into its own continuum, doctors become providers of veterinary health care services rather than managers of hospitals, and risk is diversified. These four factors arise from and influence the mission, vision, values, goals and objectives, and expectations for the merger evolution.

THE FUNCTIONING MODELS

There are many hospital affiliation or merger models operating, but they are virtually all in human health care. The simplest merger concept is that providers, facilities, and financial systems come together to deliver quality health care. In the early 1980s, hospitals formed holding companies and gave limited authority to a primary board that operated through multiple levels of management oversight at multiple facilities. No one wanted to give up control. In the later part of the 1980s, the holding companies evolved to parent companies with increased authority and a more consolidated board structure but also multiple management teams and diversified accountabilities. Control became centralized. In the early 1990s, a system orientation with central authority replaced the parent company, most often with a single board and single management

---

Box 2: Reality check

Although most well-managed mature practices can operate at 9% to 15% true net (after equitable salaries, reasonable rent, and an appropriate return on investment to the investors), in merged practices, we see a 6% to 14% increase in the individual practice net when the books must be kept squeaky clean.

In a succession planning sequence, one must clean up bookkeeping at least 5 years before retirement to maximize the sale return.

team. The "system" had multiple hospitals and other ancillary health care associated units to capitalize upon the economies of scale available to the evolving group. Many permeations of these styles of merger models are applicable to veterinary medicine. The precipitating factor is that inevitable evolution cannot be stopped but can be guided. What has also become evident is that almost all merger processes can be categorized into four phases. These definitive phases can be illustrated in a merger "Process Flow Model" (Table 1).

Anxiety is common to the initial awareness of the merger or affiliation need as well as the implementation of the merger. Phases I and II are generally initiated without a consultant if the four basic "Harvard Rules of Negotiation" are followed: (1) discuss interests but not positions; (2) separate the people from the issues; (3) seek creative solutions; and (4) above all else, apply objective criteria to operational concerns. My fifth rule of an affiliation, merger, or buy-sell is as follows: do not discuss or even guess at a price until after a valuation is completed, hopefully, by a veterinary-savvy valuation expert who uses the 12 risk factors established by the AVPMCA. Stating a price without adequate foundation knowledge of its actual value has destroyed many a potential buy-sell.

As the key players enter phase III, generally, an objective and independent arbitrator will be required to champion the merger outcome. Phase III includes definition of the mission, clarity of vision, identification of goals and objectives, physical and operational structure planning, power and control issues, and standards of care, and climaxes with conflict resolution and a "letter of intent" between the key players. Phase IV often requires the consultant but in some cases can be facilitated by a new hospital administrator hired by all of the key players to ensure the merger outcome is successful. Phase IV explores the opportunity quantifications, business plan development, task force

Table 1 Process flow model					
Phase	**I**	**II**	**III**	**IV**	**V**
Situation awareness (anxiety)	Partner assessment and selection	Initial partner discussion	Relationship concepts and $ agreements	Concept development and diligence	Implementation (anxiety)
Vision[a]	Core values[b]	Mission focus[c]	Standards of care[d]	Stair-step stock purchase[e]	Transition consultant

[a] The 5- to 10-year goal from the practice stated so clearly that everyone believes, and is so motivational, that coming back to the planned track is embraced by all.

[b] Inviolate beliefs that all team members know can be used for unilateral problem solving and project management.

[c] Internal to the practice, applying to all programs and services, to ensure it meets the vision and core values as well as the standards of care (unlike the mission statement, which usually includes the role in the community).

[d] A set of expectations for consistent quality veterinary health care delivery, embracing the best technology and products available.

[e] A tailored system that allows the buyer to purchase small affordable percentages of the practice over time.

interface, organization model, and actual merger documents that must precede the implementation. There are four basic merger models, which range from greater autonomy to more centralized control (Fig. 1).

OPERATIONAL CONCERNS DURING MERGERS

The legal entity of the merger could be a C corporation, S corporation, a limited liability company (LLC), or some other emerging structure. It varies by state or province; therefore, one should seek legal assistance from a qualified attorney with experience in professional health care legal entities. Again, there are some loose guidelines, such as keeping the land and building outside the merged practice entity, although there may initially be common players in both groups. Over time, the merged practice will want to sell small shares of the practice to allow a continuous ownership transfer to become the standard. The land and building may become assets of an estate. It does not matter when the practice is separated and operated as its own entity. If in doubt during phase I or II considerations, try to determine who owns the human health care facility in your community and how the local human hospital board is configured. Learn from those who have already done it.

The control of the new entity is vested in a "governance board," sometimes a large group as with an emergency hospital, but more often in practice mergers (specialty groups or general practices) in a smaller group, with a very basic one practice–one vote (governance is discussed in greater detail in the text *Veterinary Management in Transition: Preparing for the 21st Century*) [7]. The central issues of governance boards revolve around the questions of who, when, and how in succession and risk management situations. Once the board is established, the management philosophy must follow, including medical director authority, CEO requirements, the new hospital administrator position, the degree of board involvement in daily operations (the less the better), and the new community profile.

The clinical and nonclinical consolidation of people, supplies, and equipment sounds far easier than it ever really will be. The professional staff will become merged, as will the paraprofessional staff, and these people must deal with daily health care delivery concerns. How will the new entity build on the existing human resource strengths? What effect will historical relationships play? What is the commitment level of each player? Can they meet the most economic integration efforts planned by the new hospital administrator? How

```
                    Autonomy Centralized Control
         ┬              ┬              ┬              ┬
     Network         Joint         Holding         Merged
    Affiliation    Operating       Company        Operating
                    Company                       Corporation
```

Fig. 1. Merger models.

will the traditional senior players feel when their original practice control mechanisms are eliminated (which is a requirement for success)? These issues will all be complicated by nonroutine capital expenses, such as a new computer and fiscal management system for the merged entity.

After phase I and phase II discussions, the search for the champion of the outcome may be the most critical element of the merger process. There must be a common trust by all players. If all of the players are not ready to compromise for the new entity, do not start the process. Realign the players so that those who remain are willing to release personal control and to compromise for the good of the community and the new veterinary health care entity. Then start over. You can win!

PRACTICE VALUATION

You have done every thing to build a viable expansive practice with people excited about the quality of medicine provided and the knowledge that you are the standard in your community and among your colleagues. Now you look ahead and wonder just what you have built. What is your practice worth in the cold morning light of the marketplace?

The simplest answer is also the most complex. An accountant will tell you the value of your practice is the sum of the assets and the net earnings that result from the exercise of the assets. Then he or she will tell you the street value of the building, the equipment, the cash, and the inventory. She or he will also tell you the amount of money left over last year when all of the legitimate and reasonable expenses are paid and can also be sold (given the correct conditions, period of transition, economic conditions of the community, competition from your beloved colleagues), leading you to say, "Whoa back, mule. What about good will?"

My colleague Dr. Rob Deegan, also a valuation specialist, replies as follows: "And he/she says, quietly, looking you right in your steely-gray lights, 'There is no Goodwill.' And the CPA is not smiling. And you realize that the world doesn't take heed of the twenty years you spent 80 hours a week building the practice. Because a buyer won't care. All that counts is what you actually did for your time, how you did it, and what net did your business show each year in the recent past."

Although the practice value is based on the cold hard logic of "the money talking," the steps you took to get to the place you are will determine what you have. All those years what "they" were telling you was wrong. The assets you have in the practice of medicine based on the three P's of asset assessment are as follows:

> **Practice place.** This asset comprises all equipment and the facility, which will show up as a line item in the practice valuation.
> **People.** This asset is all of the staff—the veterinarians, the paraprofessionals, and the other support staff down to and including maintenance and animal caretakers. As you know, these are the only kinds of people you have working for you, as discussed in the trilogy *Building the Successful Veterinary*

Practice [8]. Plus, those pesky clients, dare we say they are your most valuable and vital asset. You bet!

Posterity. How hard did you look to the future? How heavily did you invest in your dreams and the dreams of your compatriots? It is going to show up every day in the operations of the practice (eg, the outpatient nurse technicians who translate your gross into practice net, those who convert a good diagnosis into quality patient care, those who increase surveillance of any deferred or symptomatic care case, those who convert your practice philosophy into active follow-up of recall, recheck, and remind).

The picture that emerges of the practice value hinges on the effective use and potentiation of the resources: human, capital, and material. How has the practice promoted training and how has it expanded the role of all staff? How has the practice supported the individual growth of knowledge and skills? How has attitude been maintained? The environment of the health care delivery system influences the practice value. If the owner has disengaged and carries a minor caseload, the practice is usually worth more than that of the veterinarian who still controls everything and does the major share of the workload. It is easier to transition when clients are bonded to the practice rather than to a single doctor.

All of the past resource use shows up on the valuation, but the value develops quietly for a long time before most practitioners want to ask for it back. Most owners do not even understand their own balance sheet. A review of the valuation concepts in the AVPMCA 12 risk factors (http://www.avpmca.org) will reveal how the factors of leadership, management, and quality health care delivery figure into the equation.

THE VALUE OF THE PRACTICE IS THE SUM OF TANGIBLE ASSETS, CLIENT RECORDS, AND THE NET EXCESS EARNINGS

The first asset on the list is real estate. The practice may actually own the land and building, but, more often, veterinarians (for good reason) own the building outside of the fiscal practice structure. If they do, the practice has a leasehold improvement asset that depreciates over time, and the practice has rent instead of a mortgage. The practice real estate needs a professional appraisal on a timely basis, which is subject to the swings of the local economy. Do not guess on this and ensure that the appraiser understands that a veterinary practice is, by necessity, the best use of a veterinary facility.

Inside the building are the bits, pieces, and tools of the trade. This equipment is essential to the operation of the practice and comes in a wide variety of ages and quality (Box 3). The most honest value of the equipment is its replacement value or the cost to get another piece of equipment to do the same job. Because the preowned equipment market has escalated in the new millennium, values are easier to ascertain. Records can be used to arrive at this figure, or a knowledgeable and profession-specific individual can be hired. The critical issue is the purpose of assessing the value. If the value will be used for a sale outside the practice, there needs to be a more rigorous and definable process. For internal

> ### Box 3: Valuation of equipment
>
> A piece of equipment may be so old that you cannot get another like it, or none of the newer generation equipment bothers to perform that task (a clue that your medical skills need attention). If there is no replacement, there is probably no value.
>
> Another consideration is how much life there is left in a piece of equipment. It is necessary to discount the replacement value according to its expected longevity. Consider a value of 60% on equipment over 2 years old that is subject to rapid wear, tear, and obsolescence. Equipment without moving parts, made of stainless steel, and having a reputation for a long life is often worth almost 80% of the original value.

use among consenting adults, as is true for a partnership or other practice management issues, jointly establishing an internal value is appropriate.

In addition to the equipment, there is inventory (Box 4). These entities are the consumable supplies ranging from paper towels to antibiotics to set-ups for the blood chemistry machine. The practice inventory control program, either computerized or hand maintained, will give a close approximation of the value (no system = minimal value). Often, a simple "touch-each-thing" count is need for valuation. If the practice is complying with taxation requirements, a wall-to-wall inventory of all expendable property is conducted at least annually to check on the flow of materials.

Frequently, all or some of the above assets have an attached liability in the form of a debt, mortgage, lease, or loan. A liability is a tool of business, as discussed previously, and is not to be shunned. Although debt may be as dangerous as a scalpel in a kindergartener's paw, it is also a thing of beauty and art in the hand of a surgeon. Of interest is the long-term amount of principal due. The current cost, both interest and current principal, is a matter of expense.

The most notable and observable asset is cash. This asset, or the lack of it, is the primary cause of practitioners berating their accountants or calling on consultants. Cash may be sitting in a bank account or a short-term note. It may be in a Mason jar in the biologics refrigerator. It may be on the books as accounts receivable (the tax man likes this asset, so keep it small) with a modest discount for the deadbeat fringe who will not pay (less than 1% annual write-off is an acceptable tolerance). Cash also has its own liability set-off, called accounts payable.

Your valuable clients (all of them) can be quantified using higher mathematics such as adding, subtracting, and multiplying. The client who gives you

> ### Box 4: Valuation of inventory
>
> Inventory has a maximum value for about 6 months. The economic turnover in this economy precludes holding on to consumables any longer. Count anything older than 6 months as a value of zero. Use it or lose it!

more business in a year is fiscally more significant to your practice than the one who comes in every third year for Fluffy's rabies vaccination; however, no single client can be quantified in monetary terms. This important fact must be remembered. The most important client you have is the one you look at every day—your staff!

For the purpose of valuation statistics, you can characterize your client base and assign a value to the entire base. The factors that apply here are the average client transaction, the retention rate of clients in your practice, the 1-year present value of future earnings, the "class of return rate" for the client base, and the number of clients in each class.

One additional measurement of the practice value is the net excess earnings. The assets are static on their own. How the practice uses the assets determines whether the practice entity remains operational, performing quality medicine and providing peace of mind to many people. After all the bills are paid and equipment replaced as needed, there is a measurement called "profit." This value is frequently given different names and measured differently under different circumstances (so buyer beware). A practice owner may have one number for his or her buddies at the American Veterinary Medicine Association (AVMA) convention and yet another for the IRS. The difference is often found in the "art" of practice valuation.

An innovative and creative accountant is a good thing, but this person needs to work for the practice and not just their computer. The first report generated in the valuation process should be the practice's cash flow situation. A sole owner may feel that his or her profit is what is left over after everybody else is paid. This owner may hold title to the real estate under a private mortgage. This structure is fine for daily operations; however, when the practice has to pay all clinicians' salaries and rent and provide reasonable operating expense monies, the formula becomes clouded. What is left after people and overhead are paid, regardless of how the accountant reports the cash flow, is the true "net profit," called net excess earnings. This amount is often confused with the return on investment, but, again, different accountants may calculate this differently. Do not let them confuse the numbers beyond the understanding of the ownership. The net excess earnings is the money left over after everything else is paid. It is the money available for reinvestment or the payoff of liabilities. It is the money a new owner would have to pay the debt of practice procurement. This amount is the measure of the financial success of the practice.

We have encountered a practice with close to $800,000 in gross sales but only $14,000 in excess earnings. Consider this statement closer—the practice is doing business but has only $14,000 at the end of the year to reinvest. This situation is an extreme example but it is not alone in our experience. This practice entity, in effect, has an approximated value of only $39,000, not much compared with the value of the assets, and the size of the gross is moot. To reiterate, the value of the practice is the "value of the assets" plus the "net excess earnings" of the practice over a measurable near future.

SUCCESSION PLANNING SUMMARY

This article has been a long and laborious discussion of something most veterinary practice owners delay in assessing. There are a half-dozen "essential" attributes to being a savvy practice owner, which allow for easier succession planning:

- He or she develops a clear vision, inviolate core values, and a consistent standard of care to support the mission focus and continuity of care between providers.
- He or she embraces team-based health care delivery models, including a proactive approach to wellness surveillance and the AVMA's "Think Twice For Life" initiative (http://www.npwm.com).
- He or she is always looking for the successor in every associate hired. Hiring warm bodies is no longer a profitable decision.
- He or she uses an established veterinary chart of accounts and follows the procedure counts as well as the financial position of the practice.
- He or she has a solid business team behind the scenes, including a veterinary-savvy attorney, a veterinary-aware CPA, a personal banker, a veterinary-specific consultant, and an investment advisor.
- He or she has the practice valued every 2 years for stock value as well as insurance purposes. The changes in practice value should reflect the increases in net income.

"Live long and prosper!"—Spock, Star Trek

References

[1] Tucker RB. Managing the future. (ISBN 0-399-13576-6).
[2] Building the successful veterinary practice: innovation & creativity, vol. 3. Blackwell Press.
[3] AVMA Directory 2005. p. 100.
[4] Building the successful veterinary practice: programs & procedures, vol. 2. Blackwell Press.
[5] CENSHARE. The pet connection. University of Minnesota.
[6] Beyond the successful veterinary practice: succession planning & other legal issues. Blackwell Press.
[7] Veterinary management in transition: preparing for the 21st century, chapter 2. Blackwell Press.
[8] Building the successful veterinary practice. Blackwell Press.

ELSEVIER
SAUNDERS

Vet Clin Small Anim 36 (2006) 373–384

VETERINARY CLINICS
SMALL ANIMAL PRACTICE

Buying and Leasing Real Estate for Veterinary Hospitals

Karl R. Salzsieder, DVM, JD

Salzsieder Consulting and Legal Services, 611 Cowlitz Way West, Suite B, Kelso WA 98626, USA

OVERVIEW

Real estate costs or rent expenses include the building and land lease costs paid to an outside party or to the owner of the practice (if the building is owned separately from the business). They do not include mortgage payments or the interest portion of a mortgage [1]. These costs are a major part of the expenses of any veterinary hospital business operation. This is true whether the real estate is purchased by the prospective practice owner or whether it is leased. If the practice facility is leased, the lease costs, as part of the operations expenses, in a well-managed practice should run 5% on a triple net basis or between 6% and 8% of the total gross revenue if you include property taxes, insurance, and utilities, which make up the triple net costs.

Keep in mind that these statistics are for "well-managed practices" [2]. You might expect their revenue to be higher or their square footage smaller for more efficiency to decrease the rent costs percentage. If you look at rent expense as a percentage of total income from a much broader base of practices, the rent expense averages 6.6%, and this average varies by region, metro status, number of veterinarians, and total income [1].

The average practice in the West reported a rent expense of 6.9%, which is significantly higher than the average practice in the Northeast (5.3%). Urban practices also reported a significantly higher average (7.1%) than rural practices (5.7%). Practices with more than two veterinarians have a lower rent expense at 5.4% than practices with two or fewer veterinarians [2].

Depending on the terms and the down payment, if any, when the practitioner becomes a real estate purchaser, the costs (in terms of contract or mortgage payments) are usually less than lease expenses. Of course, this could vary with the amount of the purchase price of the property, the interest rate, and the amount of down payment made by the purchaser.

If one looks only at the real estate costs as the mortgage payment, including principal and interest (from a 2001 calendar year survey) [1], the average amount spent as a percentage of total income is 6.5%. Again, these percentages

E-mail address: karl@vetbizlaw.com

0195-5616/06/$ – see front matter
doi:10.1016/j.cvsm.2005.10.007

vary with location, number of veterinarians, and gross revenue of the practice [1]. The highest percentage is 7.0% for the metro and suburban practices.

Again, these percentages do not include the triple net type lease expenses of insurance, taxes, and utilities. These costs are usually passed along to the tenant as operating costs. Therefore, if one took out the principal payment part of the mortgage payment, the payment would be much smaller, but without knowing the variables cited previously, this is not possible.

Also, as mentioned elsewhere in this article, some leases to veterinary practices may be submarket because of non–third-party owners or because the practice real estate is not used for the highest and best use for its location.

When analyzing the percentage of revenue for real estate costs, whether from a lease or from a mortgage payment, the tenant should realize that these costs are likely to be higher for a new start-up practice or for a practice that has recently enlarged its space or recently built or purchased a new facility. In these cases, the practice may still have to grow into the expanded physical plant.

The author has seen practices, after moving into a new facility, where the mortgage payments initially may reach 12% to 18% of the practice's gross revenue. These practices usually have plans to grow into the new expanded hospital area, knowing and expecting the temporary higher facility costs (as a percentage of revenue) to lower as the practice grows and the revenue increases, while the facility costs remain near constant over time, except for the market appreciation variations that may affect lease payments or the interest rate changes that may affect the mortgage payments. The core question is whether to lease or to purchase the real estate.

In decision making, when purchasing a veterinary practice or planning to expand the current facility, whether with remodeling or with a total new construction, one of the big questions is whether or not the practice owner should be purchasing or leasing the real estate portion of the practice.

In the 2002 American Animal Hospital Survey of 882 respondents, 77% reported that they owned rather than rented their facility. Also, that survey confirmed that in practices of one or fewer veterinarians, 82% owned, whereas only 74% of those surveyed owned if there were more than two veterinarians.

Contrary to common knowledge, practices that are merely expanding by remodeling or practices that are building a totally new building can, like a new practice purchaser, still have a third party own the expanded or new facility and lease it back for the practice use if they desire [3].

If a practice is being sold, most real estate–owning practice sellers would prefer to hold the real estate and lease it to the new practice purchaser. This gives the seller a longer stream of income, which is secured by the real estate. The seller is usually happy with selling the practice and leasing the real estate, because new practice owners are good long-term tenants in most cases, who provide the real estate owner with stability and longevity for his or her investment. Also, new practice owners presumably pay the real estate owner a market rate of rent.

Most noncorporate practice purchasers would rather purchase the real estate. This is especially true when all other issues are equal and cash for the down payment is not an issue. This is to assist in decreasing the practice's lease expense item, assuming that the building purchaser agrees to make the mortgage payment be equal to the lease payment charged to the practice and that the real estate purchase price is not unusually high.

Most corporate practice purchasers do not purchase practice real estate (personal interview with three major corporate executives–Scott Campbell, DVM, CEO, Banfield, 2000; Stan Creighton, CEO, National Veterinary Association, 2004; and Michael Everett, JD, Corporate Counsel, Veterinary Centers of America, 2004). The reasons for both sides of this issue are explored in this article.

DEFINITIONS

Renting and *leasing* are terms that are commonly used interchangeably and refer to different terms of a contract to use and control a facility by paying the landlord, usually monthly or annually, for the use of the facility. Technically, renting or having a rental contract refers to paying to use a facility for less than a year. A lease contract is to provide for paying for the use and control of a facility for a period of 1 year or longer. Most leases are drafted to be triple net leases. This requires the tenant to pay most repairs and maintenances as well as taxes, insurance, and utilities.

Most lease terms in the business arena are for a period of 3 to 5 years. Most lenders want the lease to be for a minimum of 7 to 10 years or at least for the total period of pay-back time for any business financing. To allow flexibility to the practice purchaser, one should use the 3- to 5-year lease with several additional lease options as needed.

Options to renew the lease are short agreements, usually incorporated in the lease, to allow a tenant to commit to leasing for a shorter time initially (still for a minimum of 1 to 3 or 5 years) but still to have the discretion to renew (or not) the initial lease for one or more similar periods.

In most cases, the author's advice for leasing is to secure the facility by obtaining a lease for the shortest period the landlord agrees to (usually from 1 to 3 years) and then to include (in the lease) a number of lease options to renew (for 3 to 5 years each) as needed for meeting the term of years that the lender requires.

The use of a short-term lease with several options to renew allows the tenant (eg, practitioner, owner of the business) to have flexibility if an issue comes up regarding the health of the practitioner or the health of the business. There may also be issues regarding the facility or its location. Of course, the landlord is likely to request and prefer a longer term single-period lease to be able to have stability in tenancy.

The main disadvantage for the tenant in having shorter lease periods with several lease options to renew is that it may allow for more frequent escalations of the lease price. The landlord may sometimes raise the lease price at each option exercise period.

Most leases ordinarily have annual lease price escalation clauses in the original lease document. If the cost of living should increase more than predicted in
the initial lease escalation clause, however, the shorter term lease with the option to renew would allow the landlord to make those needed adjustments to
the lease price.

If the practice owner also owns the facility, the leasing entity would then be
the practitioner (business owner), which could be set up as a proprietorship or
as a separate real estate business entity. In almost all cases, it is recommended
that a separate real estate business entity be set up to be the real estate owner
and landlord; then, a different and separate business entity is the veterinary
practice tenant, even if the principal of both entities is the same owner or
owners.

Most third-party landlords agree to lease to a veterinary practice that is set
up as a separate business entity, but they may also require the shareholders
be personal guarantors for the lease. This is a common acceptable practice as
long as the practice business entity has terms in its documentation to allow
for the guarantors to be indemnified should there be some loss that would
pass to the guarantors.

In the past, there were a lot of sole owners set up as proprietorships or partnerships as business owners. Today, with the increasing risk of liability for veterinary practice owners, the veterinary practice business, in almost all cases,
should be a separate entity that is not a proprietorship or partnership and
not the owner of the real estate. The real estate ownership should be a separate
business entity, which is neither a proprietorship nor a partnership.

If one goes beyond the proprietorship and partnership for the real estate
ownership, the main entity options are the corporation and the limited liability
company (LLC). In most states, the veterinary business LLC would really be
set up as a professional limited liability company (PLLC), whereas the real estate entity would be an LLC.

With the increasing acceptance of the LLC, most new business formations,
whether for practice businesses or for real estate ownership, are LLCs if the
company is not planning to go to public ownership later by selling regulated
securities on a stock exchange.

There are a few real estate ownership corporations or real estate investment
trusts (REITS), which can be small private ownership companies or publicly
traded companies, depending on how many owners there are. Currently, for
small real estate businesses, the trend is to have the real estate–owning entity
be an LLC. This organization has the liability protection of a corporation
but requires less formality for shareholder meetings and minutes, for example.
There is not space, nor is it the purpose of this article, to go into all the reasons
to choose one entity over another; however, in most cases, the author recommends an LLC as the business entity, whether for the business or for the real
estate ownership.

Purchasing the real estate may be easier than a novice investor might think.
Most lenders would prefer that a practice purchaser buy the real estate

whenever there is a sufficient down payment to meet the lender's requirement. This allows the practice lender to combine security not only in the practice but in the real estate.

One source of down payment (as far as the lender is concerned) is for the seller to agree to take a carry-back note to be recorded after the financing is completed with the bank. This means that the seller would have to be subordinate or in second place as far as security in the real estate is concerned.

That allows the lender to be in first place in the real estate security. With this scenario, the lender can treat the seller's financing (carry-back note) as he or she would a purchaser's down payment in regard to the loan-to-value ratio for the real estate. Most lenders only lend up to 75% or 80% of the value of the real estate. Therefore, if the purchaser did not have the 20% to 25% down payment, the seller could carry that amount as a note subordinate to the lender in the form of a carry-back note, as described previously. The only other limiting factor is that some lenders also have operating procedures that require a minimum investment with cash from the purchaser. There are also some lenders, however, who (if the loan to value ratio is covered as described previously) are willing to lend to the purchaser to the level of essentially having 100% financing or nothing down.

"To purchase or to lease the real estate" is a question that goes beyond the purchaser down payment issue. The analysis is found in the review of the landlord investor's expected return or return on investment (ROI) calculations and comparing those with the minimum real estate contract or mortgage payment schedules, including today's interest rates.

Some consultants or advisors would also advocate, if the veterinary tenant's business ROI is high enough (greater than the normal real estate investment ROI), that one should consider the opportunity costs of not owning more or other like kind veterinary practice businesses instead of having equity in the real estate [3]. This author believes that this opportunity cost theory consideration, other than for large corporations with the mission to expand almost without limit, is not an issue for most practices in the small veterinary practice business model.

This is especially true when the National Commission on Veterinary Economic Issues (NCVEI) continues to show the average net return (ROI) after practitioner compensation and rent expenses and operating expenses for the veterinary practice business to range between only 5% and 7%. Any prospective veterinary real estate buyer should realize that well-managed veterinary practices receive a practice return (ROI) of 11.8% [2].

Real estate investors in most states expect a minimum of 8.5% to 10% net return on their investment (ROI) [4]. This expected investment return is calculated on the real estate purchase price or on the fair market value of the real estate as of the lease execution date and annually thereafter. Some investors and historical rules of thumb have stated that the lease rate for the specialty single-use veterinary practice real estate should be 1% per month or 12% per year of the fair market value. This would be at the high end, in unique markets, or for mature well-managed practices.

With any of these ROI rates affecting the lease rate, the reader can understand that if a real estate purchaser can borrow the real estate purchase funds at 6% to 7% or even slightly higher, the cash flow would be expected to be less than leasing, even knowing that the mortgage payments would include some small amount for principal payments.

Of course, the income tax effect for the cash outflow regarding the lease versus the purchase payment would be different. This is because the lease payments are 100% tax-deductible expenses to the business entity but the mortgage payments would only include the interest portion as a tax-deductible expense to the business entity [1]. The Internal Revenue Service (IRS) tax code prevents real estate purchasers from declaring mortgage principal payments from being an operating expense, thus not a tax-savings expense.

With real estate of any reasonable size, where the construction costs without the land can be in the range of $125 to $160 per square foot, it is easy to realize that a hospital in even the relatively small 2000–sq ft size, including the land, would be in the price range of $300,000 to $350,000 for fair market value; thus, the rent could easily be in the range of $2500 to $3000 per month, whereas the payments to purchase (a total cost facility, including the land for $300,000) would be $2120.34 per month at 7% for 25 years. Here, there may be a savings of more than $800 per month if purchasing instead of leasing. Of course, this again assumes that the real estate owner (especially if also being the practice owner) charges the practice rent equal to and not greater than the mortgage payment.

Of course, these sample terms would change in an environment that included the lender's mortgage rates escalating. At present, the author is involved in consulting for several practice sales transactions, and the lenders tend to offer the purchaser mortgage money at prime plus 1% to 2%. The fixed term for these interest rates varies from 1 to 5 or 10 years before requiring an interest rate adjustment, a balloon payment for payoff, or refinancing of the remaining balance. Of course, any refinancing, like any lease renewal, would allow the lender to raise the interest rates.

This sample calculation does not estimate the federal tax savings for the real estate purchaser by his being able to depreciate the building value (not including the land value) over 39 years as a non–cash-operating expense write off. This tax savings is in addition to the interest and cash expense, while, usually at the same time, accruing a real estate noncash appreciation of 3% to 7% or more per year, depending on the location of the property. Most long-term comparisons of average real estate appreciation rates indicate that an annual appreciation rate of at least 3% is reasonable [2].

Some locations in the United States have periodic appreciation rates as high as 7% to 12% or more in a year [2]. The real estate appreciation is a noncash benefit that cannot be realized by the real estate owner until the time of sale of the property. This real estate sale usually does not happen until the time of sale of the practice unless there is a practice move before or concurrent with the practice sale. Of course, these real estate ownership benefits are not available for the strip center type practices that are not free standing, where a lease is the only vehicle to allow the practice owner to be in control and in use of the real estate.

Another benefit that favors real estate ownership is the frequent easy financing. Lenders tend to view real estate as having an almost unlimited lifespan as compared with their view of other capital investments used in the business operation.

The converse to the easy borrowing opportunity for real estate purchasing is the risk that the interest rates from the lenders may rise faster than a comparable period lease escalation factor would, thus raising the effective net cost of owning beyond the gradual increases in the lease alternative. If the purchaser of real estate can afford some interest fluctuation, the added benefit of the appreciation mentioned previously may still make it worthwhile to purchase rather than to lease the real estate.

In summary, the major factors to be considered in the real estate purchase decision are the interest rate, the depreciation schedule, the property appreciation, the income tax impact, and the impact of paying a principal payment as part of the real estate mortgage. All these factors must be compared with the costs of leasing.

Leasing real estate beyond an analytical approach to the lease document itself really only involves the term (period of lease agreement), the price, and the lease options to extend, plus any landlord-provided improvement allowances for remodeling or for property interior design change.

These tenancy improvement allowances are usually only available for a start-up practice that might be moving into a strip center type facility. Here, the landlord may offer the practitioner(s) as a move-in incentive a $2 to $3 per square foot financial incentive to assist in the finish work and design as chosen by the prospective tenant. Sometimes, if the leasable space is in a newly constructed site, the allowance may be much greater to the first tenant. This can be up to $5 per square foot or more. Here, there may be some items of internal construction that have not yet been completed, and the tenant is required to complete them with some of the move-in allowance.

The final purchase analysis, other than a review of the documents themselves and a review of the property itself, really involves the purchaser's ability to finance and the opportunity costs of the business, if any. With veterinary practice average net earnings currently being relatively low, as mentioned previously, in comparison with other businesses, the opportunity costs for investing more in the practice versus making the investment in the real estate may be insignificant. This author believes that the results point in the direction of real estate ownership, unless a specific practice has the benefit of being one of a few of the exceptionally well-managed practices that may be building net earnings around 12% or up to an occasional 17% to 20% of the gross revenue.

In these practices, the practice owners must assess the cost benefits of taking money that could be invested in the real estate and determining if those same dollars added to the practice would continue to generate the same higher rate of return. If that answer is yes, before investing additional dollars in real estate, the practice owners may do better to invest those same dollars in more earning assets for the practice.

Assuming the final real estate decision is to lease, to assist a potential veterinary practice owner in procuring and completing a real estate lease, what follows are the main points that a veterinary practice tenant must cover in a lease document. These are ideas from the author's legal documents.

The lease document should be variable in length, up to 25 to 30 pages, depending on the drafter. One main issue that must be covered is the naming of the landlord, the naming of the tenant, and their associated entities. The lease must have the address of the premises. It should refer to other related agreements that may be relative to this lease. Of course, that includes reference to any purchase and sale agreements on the practice if the tenant was concurrently a new practice purchaser.

The commencement date for the effectiveness of the lease should be listed. The term must be listed. This can vary from 1 year to 3 or 5 years or 10 to 20 years. If the term is reasonably short, less than 5 years, there may also be a listing about the number of renewal terms or options to renew that the tenant may have discretion to exercise. There needs to be an explanation of the length of each renewal term and the associated rent.

The lease must include the base rent terms and escalation clauses. Commonly, the lease lists a given year, the annual base rent, and the monthly base rent. Some strip center type leaseholds include a percentage of the revenue of the practice, and they may have a requirement for contribution to advertising expenses that are incurred on behalf of all tenants of the strip center. It is recommended these percentage revenue and advertising expenses be eliminated if possible.

The lease should include any additional charges that are to be paid by the tenant. These additional charges could include maintenance of the facility, real estate taxes of the facility, and casualty insurance of the facility, all of which may be part of the triple net fees. Other issues regarding parking of customers and tenants of the leasehold premises are also important.

Other associated documents could include the right of first refusal to purchase or an option to purchase the building. The lease should include the premises area, the leasehold premises square foot area, and if in a strip center, that square foot space as compared with total center's leasable space. This is needed to allow for proration dividing of the expenses of the common areas to each tenant.

The lease should include statements about prepayments. Commonly, the tenant must pay the first and last month's rent in advance plus a damage deposit, which may or may not equal 1 month's rent. The lease should discuss triple net fees, which are now most common for tenants to pay, even though if in a center, it would be the tenant's proportionate share of the expenses for taxes, insurance, and maintenance costs, plus management fees.

Some of the areas mentioned previously that may be negotiable before signing a lease include the following:

1. The premise's square footage, depending on the location of the facility and whether or not it is in a center
2. The original term, in which it is usually preferable to the tenant that shorter term leases exist with several options to renew
3. The base rent should be within reason even though it is tied to the market rate. The market rate is negotiable, however, because there are differences in location, quality, and maintenance levels of different buildings. Part of the rate issue would be whether or not the adjacent properties are fully occupied or vacant and where the community is for this facility versus where the market rent surveys have come from.
4. The tenant is to pay the taxes and assessments regarding the real estate. This can be handled by the tenant paying these taxes directly or by the landlord paying the taxes and requesting the tenant for reimbursement. Sometimes, it is worthwhile to negotiate this issue, because some commercial leases include a 5% to 10% management fee if the landlord is involved in paying these assessments and requesting reimbursements. It may be negotiable to save the management fee if the tenant agrees to pay these taxes and assessments directly.
5. Likewise with insurance, the tenant may discover that a lower limit of liability saves a reasonably large amount of money. The landlord usually wants the limits of liability to be higher to prevent a concurrent law suit in the case of loss against the landlord if the tenant's insurance was not large enough, however. Again, there may be some savings if the tenant agrees, if possible, to get his or her own insurance without having it processed by the landlord to save the management fee assessment.
6. The tenant, especially in a free-standing facility, agrees to pay his or her own utilities, including gas, electric, water, telephone, and any other utilities on the premises. If the facility is in a center, the landlord may have to do a proportionate assessment of the sum or all of these fees, depending on the metering in the facility.
7. The maintenance costs of the facility can again be a tenant's obligation or a landlord's obligation, depending on the location of the facility and whether or not there are other tenants sharing these costs. If the facility is free standing, it is suggested the tenant take full responsibility for maintenance to save management costs and, possibly, to allow some control of quality and quantity. Another important maintenance issue that has to do with the itemization of expenses for the tenant is the costs for the heating, ventilation, and air-conditioning (HVAC) systems. These systems are expensive to replace. If a tenant should occupy a facility that has other than new equipment still under warranty, the tenant could be liable or responsible in the first year of tenancy to have to replace an HVAC unit, which could run from $5000 to $20,000 depending on the size of the unit. This particular topic must be negotiated. If the tenant is responsible for replacing this capital expense item, repayment can be spread over several years for repayment. Alternately, it may be negotiated that the landlord is responsible 100% for the first 1 or 2 years of the lease.

8. If the tenant does not have a long-term historic perspective on the triple net costs (including insurance, taxes, and maintenance), he or she should negotiate for an annualized maximum triple net fee to protect himself or herself from being overly assessed.

9. Alterations issues are important for a tenant to negotiate, particularly if the tenant plans more than interior decorating changes to the facilities. Commonly, if this is a new practice purchase-related real estate transaction, the landlord may even provide $2 to $3 or more per square foot for the tenant to use for changing the interior of the facility.

10. The lease should provide for casualty loss and whether or not the landlord can evict the tenant, depending on the percentage of the space that is damaged. This again can be negotiated, depending on the tenant's willingness to tolerate inconvenience and mess should there be a fire or other damage.

11. There should be a provision clarifying that the landlord does not allow the tenant to cause any attachment to the premises for any lien for work done. Nevertheless, there must be an exception in that lien section that does allow the tenant to have the right at any time to grant a security interest in any goods and property that the tenant owns.

12. A section should set parking regarding the location of vehicles for the tenant's employees, which is usually a separate space from the parking area for the tenant's customers.

13. There should be a provision for surrender of the premises describing the conditions and fixtures that may be left or not by the tenant on departure on expiration of the lease.

14. There should be a section regarding the landlord's failure to maintain the areas of the tenancy in the landlord's absence so that the tenant can get things fixed, such as a leaky roof, if the landlord does not reasonably take remedial action, usually within 10 to 20 days.

15. The tenant has a right to quiet enjoyment, which means that the landlord does not have a right to enter, except for specific reasons.

16. There should be discussion on the title to improvements and equipment, particularly relating to trade fixtures furnished by the tenant. There should be requirements about tenant signs conforming to those of other tenancies in a center or not to harm the facility in attachment of other signs.

17. There are specific issues to be discussed about the access to the premises by the landlord and how much notice might be required or an exception for emergencies.

18. An assignment and subletting section should be negotiated so that the tenant has the right to assign the lease, particularly if the tenant agrees to sell the practice or even if the tenant decides to move and cannot break the lease at the time of moving. This would allow the tenant the right to be able to sublease the space to prohibit continued costs for nonuse.

19. There should be a governing law section explaining where the mediation, arbitration, or litigation would take place in a dispute. There should be a mediation/arbitration section explaining that the tenant and the landlord agree to have some alternate dispute resolution methods in place rather than directly going to court. Some legal sources currently say that mediation should be the first provision, followed by litigation without arbitration, because of the increased cost of arbitration; however, of course, that is up to your legal advisor.

Assuming that the final real estate decision is to purchase, the following are some important points to be included in the purchase agreement. These are taken from the author's legal documents.

Purchasing a veterinary practice facility requires the purchaser and the seller to agree in writing for the sale and purchase. This document may be termed a *purchase and sale agreement*, or it may be termed a *sale and purchase agreement*. It is not significant other than, commonly, the drafter might put his or her reference first in that title. This document names the purchasers and the sellers, whether individuals or particular separate entities.

It lists the purchase price and how it is to be paid. The document lists the closing date and the possession date, which may or may not be the same. It specifies the type of title that is to be exchanged, preferably a warranty deed. It explains the type of title insurance required by the purchaser that the seller must provide to warranty the restrictions and liens, for example, covering the real estate to be purchased. The preliminary title report allows the purchaser to review and accept or decline the purchase based on the findings in the title report. This particular section allowing the purchaser's approval of the title report can also allow the purchaser to waive restrictions, covenants, or liens against the property and accept them as they are rather than requiring the seller to clear them off before closing.

The agreement should include an inspection contingency that provides for the purchaser to have the right, personally or through other experts, to inspect the real estate for structure, location, and Environmental Protection Agency (EPA) and hazard substances issues. The purchaser should have the right to review the books, records, and lease agreements, if any.

The purchaser has the right to access, including bringing in experts that may do core drilling, soil condition inspections, or geologic surveys, for example, including any EPA and environmental inspections. Most lenders require at least a basic phase I inspection, which is mostly a research-oriented document provided by a third party explaining the historical ownership and likelihood of EPA or environmental contaminants under the soil. If this historical phase I study provides suspicion of subterranean objects, other follow-up studies may be required. The purchaser should have full right to request those studies, along with meeting any other lender's requirements as well.

There should be a personal property section that explains all the included items that go with the sale, which includes everything (eg, fixtures, antennas, curtains). In this section, it is important to consult your certified public accountant (CPA) to agree on the final values of the personal property.

There should be a section about the seller's representation and warranties, which confirms the seller's right to sell, including books and records, for example.

There should be a provision that there are no pending or threatening litigations. The document must provide for who the closing agent is. It should provide for proration of tax expenses, who shares in the escrow closing costs, and who maintains the operations and risk of loss before closing.

The document should provide for postclosing adjustments, collections, and payments, which allows for clarifying the amounts owed by the purchaser or the seller, depending on the date of closing, because that may or may not coincide with the billing anniversary dates for utilities, for example. This document should include who is the closing agent and under which venue is the governing law. Because time is of the essence, the acceptance and counteroffers have time lines that are spelled out.

Further, it is important that the purchaser go through all issues that may be a concern for the purchaser, including financing contingencies, whether for the down payment or for the total package and whether or not the real estate purchase is subject to the purchaser's first obtaining the veterinary practice.

Therefore, a purchaser can see that a purchase and sale agreement for the real estate can be drafted and signed concurrently with a practice purchase and sale agreement, both before closing, as long as several contingencies are provided for that allow the purchaser the right to cancel and get a refund of the earnest money deposit that is making the real estate purchase and sale agreement binding.

SUMMARY

The purpose of the overview of the lease versus purchase question regarding the real estate for a veterinary practice is to confirm, given today's interest rates, if the real estate purchaser and seller can agree on the down payment and if the seller will carry back financing. If such is the case, there is almost no situation (subject to the real estate price) in which the practice purchaser should not purchase the real estate to save cash flow expenses.

One exception, especially in high-value real estate areas in which a practice owner may not be able to afford to purchase the real estate, is when the landlord may not have raised the lease price over time. That is, the landlord may not have raised the lease price to get his rate of return based on the fair market value or when the landlord does not realize the highest and best use of the real estate; thus, the lease price is much less expensive than the purchase payments might be. If this opportunity turns out to be the case, the practice owner may be much better off to get a long-term lease rather than to attempt to purchase the real estate.

References

[1] Landeck E, editor. Financial and productivity pulsepoints. 2nd edition. Lakewood (CO): American Animal Hospital Association Press; 2002.
[2] Veterinary Economics. Companion animal study. Lenexa (KS): Advanstar Communications; 2003. p. 31, 33.
[3] Christian RS. American properties. Littleton (Co): American Pet Care Properties.
[4] McElroy K. The ABC's of real estate investing. New York: Warner Business Books; 2004.

Vet Clin Small Anim 36 (2006) 385–396

VETERINARY CLINICS
SMALL ANIMAL PRACTICE

Four Core Communication Skills of Highly Effective Practitioners

Jane R. Shaw, DVM, PhD

Argus Institute, Department of Clinical Sciences, College of Veterinary Medicine and Biomedical Sciences, Colorado State University, 300 West Drake Road, Fort Collins, CO 80523, USA

The importance of communication in veterinary medicine is an emerging topic, as evident in multiple influential studies published in the past 5 years. For instance, one of the six critical issues identified during focus group sessions of the KPMG LLP study [1] was that "while the scientific, technical, and clinical skills of the veterinary profession remain high, there is evidence that veterinarians lack management and communication skills necessary for success in private practice." The Brakke Management Study reported that many veterinarians are not earning up to their potential and suggested that a limiting behavior was the failure to use management practices proven to improve business performance [2]. The three management practices that demonstrated the largest potential to increase income were related to employee longevity, employee satisfaction, and client satisfaction. A primary component of these practices involves staff and client communication. A personnel decisions study identified nontechnical competencies for career success, including interpersonal competence, work and life balance, effective communication, leadership skills, and business acumen [3]. The American Animal Hospital Association (AAHA) compliance study investigated compliance with six basic health care recommendations: heartworm testing, heartworm preventative, dental prophylaxis, therapeutic diets, preanesthetic screening, and core vaccines [4]. Noncompliance ranged from 17% to 82%, and one of the primary reasons for noncompliance was not making a recommendation because of inadequate communication.

In addition to the findings of these influential studies, there have been substantial changes in the profession that affect veterinarian-client-patient communication. One of the major changes is the increasing recognition of the relationships that people may have with their companion animals [5]. When asked about their relationship with their pets, 85% of pet owners reported that they viewed their pets as family members [1]. In conjunction with this, there is a growing recognition that provision of veterinary services in a manner

E-mail address: jane.shaw@colostate.edu

0195-5616/06/$ – see front matter
doi:10.1016/j.cvsm.2005.10.009

that acknowledges the human-animal bond should lead to better outcomes for veterinary practices and their patients [1]. Appreciating the impact of animal companionship on the health and well-being of human beings creates a new dimension for veterinarians in public health. Veterinarians' responsibilities have expanded to include attending to the well-being of their clients as well as their clients' pets [5].

In a recent address, Blackwell [5] stated that today's veterinarians are faced with educated clients armed with questions and greater expectations. Veterinarians' responsibilities for addressing questions and providing client education are increased. In an increasingly litigious society, consumers are not forgiving of unprofessional services [5]. Most complaints to regulatory bodies are related to poor communication and deficient interpersonal skills [6], with breakdown in communication being a major cause of client dissatisfaction.

There is limited information in the veterinary literature on veterinarian-client-patient communication, and what is available is predominantly based on expert opinion and anecdotal information rather than on peer-reviewed scientific studies [7]. In contrast, the human medical communication literature contains a large number of empiric studies; as a result, evidence-based recommendations guide communication skills training [8]. Much can be learned from studies of physician-patient communication to inform teaching and research programs in veterinary-client-patient communication [7].

The purpose of this article is twofold: to present four core communication skills and the associated evidence and to provide support for development and implementation of the four core communication skills in clinical practice to enhance clinical outcomes. Although empiric evidence linking communication with clinical outcomes is lacking in veterinary medicine, the author hypothesizes that effective communication between veterinarians and clients is strongly associated with improved client and pet outcomes of care.

UNDERLYING PREMISES

Based on 40 years of research in human medicine, three underlying premises guide communication skills training [8]:

1. Communication is a core clinical skill essential to clinical competence, alongside physical examination, medical knowledge, and problem solving.
2. Communication is related to significant outcomes of care, including diagnostic accuracy, time management, a collaborative physician-patient relationship, patient and physician satisfaction, adherence, patient health, and malpractice risk.
3. Communication can be taught and is a series of learned skills. Communication skills can be delineated, defined, and measured, and these skills are best learned through observation, well-intentioned and descriptive feedback, repeated practice, and rehearsal of skills.

COMMUNICATION SKILLS

Communication skills are a vital component of interpersonal interactions. Three broad types of communication skills have been identified: content skills, process skills, and perceptual skills [9,10]. Content skills are what doctors communicate—the content of their questions and the information they give. Process skills relate to how doctors communicate through verbal and nonverbal methods of communication. Verbal communication is composed of what is said, in particular word choice. Nonverbal communication is the message that is communicated without the use of words and is conveyed through verbal indicators (ie, voice tone, volume, and pitch, as well as the pace of speech), facial expression, eye contact, proximity, posture, and gestures [11]. Nonverbal communication bridges the gap between what is said and what is interpreted. Perceptual skills include cognitive skills (ie, problem solving and critical reasoning) and relationship skills (ie, awareness of others, self-awareness, and personal attitudes and biases). Content, process, and perceptual skills all contribute to the overall efficacy of communication.

VETERINARIAN-CLIENT-PATIENT RELATIONSHIP

A "gold standard" does not exist for assessing veterinarian-client interactions, nor is there an accepted definition of the ideal veterinarian-client relationship. In fact, under different clinical circumstances, different models may be appropriate and effective [12]. Flexibility is of utmost importance, and the choice of communication style should be tailored to the individual client and patient [13].

In human medical practice and veterinary practice, the most common model for the physician-patient relationship is still paternalism [14]. In this model, the veterinarian dominates the medical encounter, setting the agenda and goals for the visit, and the client's voice is diminished. The content of the discussion is predominantly biomedical, and the veterinarian plays the role of guardian of the patient and acts in the client's and patient's best interest.

In contrast, it has been proposed that the optimal model for physician-patient relationships is relationship-centered care, which reflects a balance between physician paternalism and patient autonomy [14]. Relationship-centered care is characterized as a partnership in which negotiation and shared decision-making are used to take the patient's perspective into consideration. The role of the physician is as an advisor or counselor.

The term *relationship-centered care* seems to reflect the nature of the veterinarian-client-patient relationship, which is composed of the veterinarian-client relationship, the client-pet relationship, and the veterinarian-pet relationship. In veterinary medicine, relationship-centered care is characterized by a joint venture between the veterinarian and client to provide optimal care for the animal. During the process of gathering information and client education, questions and information giving include lifestyle and social issues that may influence the pet's health. Respect for the client's perspective and interests, asking for the client's opinion, recognition of the client's expertise in caring for the pet, and acknowledgment of the role the animal plays in the family's life are incorporated into all aspects of care. The communication skills presented in this article foster the development of a collaborative veterinarian-client partnership.

FOUR CORE COMMUNICATION SKILLS

Nonverbal Communication

Nonverbal communication includes all behavioral signals between interacting individuals exclusive of verbal content and occurs in several modes [8]. These behavioral signals include body language (ie, facial expressions, gestures, body position, tension, touch); spatial relationships, including the distance between the veterinarian and client and objects that may act as potential barriers to communication (ie, examination table, animal, computer, seating); paralanguage (ie, voice tone, rate, rhythm, emphasis, volume); and autonomic responses, such as flushing, blanching, tearing, sweating, and changes in breathing pattern and pupil size, which are involuntary nonverbal responses and communicate underlying emotional responses [15].

Although estimates vary, it is recognized that as much as 80% of communication is nonverbal in nature, whereas only 20% is based on verbal content [8]. Voluntary verbal communication reflects what a person is thinking and effectively communicates discrete pieces of information. Involuntary nonverbal communication tends to reflect what a person is feeling and communicates attitudes, emotions, and affect. In most cases, verbal and nonverbal communication work together to strengthen or reinforce a message; however, on occasion, nonverbal communication can contradict verbal communication. When verbal and nonverbal communication is incongruent, a mixed message is sent and the nonverbal message more accurately reflects the true feelings and is more likely to predict behavior. Miscommunication is more likely to result when nonverbal communication is lacking, such as in a telephone conversation or an electronic-mail message.

There are two areas of focus for nonverbal communication. The first is to increase sensitivity to the nonverbal cues of the client, and the second is to enhance awareness of your own nonverbal messages [8]. The tasks associated with picking up and responding to client's nonverbal messages are to enhance sensory acuity and to reflect back what you see verbally [8]. This entails heightening awareness of nonverbal communication and picking up on nonverbal cues, such as the client tearing up, breaking eye contact, looking at his or her watch, tapping his or her feet, or displaying a concerned expression. The second step is to reflect back what you see verbally (ie, "It seems like you may have some concerns about how to progress with Max's treatment"). The final step is to factor in the client's response into your next question or direction of the interaction (ie, "We have talked about a lot of options, and this can be quite overwhelming. I would be interested in hearing what questions or concerns you have at this point"). The following example illustrates the process of picking up and responding to a client's nonverbal cues.

Example

1. Pick up on the nonverbal cue (eg, client glancing at his or her watch).
2. Reflect back to the client what you see. Veterinarian: "I notice you glancing at your watch." Client: "Yes, I'm sorry. I'm in a hurry today. How long will this take?"

3. Factor the client's response into the next part of the interaction. Veterinarian: "I'll finish up his physical exam in a few minutes, and I would like to talk to you about some approaches we might take to investigate this problem further. I am wondering whether your schedule permits this discussion today or whether we should book another appointment for later in the day or tomorrow."

It is equally important to pay attention to your own nonverbal messages to ensure that verbal and nonverbal communication work together to reinforce one another [8]. Miscommunication results when verbal and nonverbal messages are contradictory. The nonverbal message usually reflects the underlying truth. Awareness of nonverbal communication is integral to establishing and maintaining a strong collaborative veterinarian-client-patient relationship. Nonverbal communication, such as making eye contact, maintaining an attentive and open body posture, establishing a closer distance, nodding and gesturing, using a caring voice tone, and displaying emotion, has been associated with enhanced patient satisfaction [16–18].

Open-Ended Questions

Open-ended questions or statements encourage the person to elaborate or to tell a story without shaping or focusing the content (ie, "Tell me how Max has been doing since his surgery") [8]. In contrast, closed questions are questions in which a specific or one-word answer is expected (ie, "Has Max been doing okay since his surgery?"). Open and closed questions are both valuable for gathering information during the clinical interview; however, they are used to achieve different goals. A funnel technique is recommended, starting with the broad open-ended questions to obtain the problem list from the client's perspective and later asking more focused specific questions to clarify details (ie, duration, frequency, further description) [8].

Open-ended inquiry can be formulated as a statement with phrases like "tell me" or "describe for me" or as a question beginning with "how" or "what" [19]. Questions that begin with "why" may be less effective, because the answer requires a justification and could elicit a defensive response from the client.

Examples
- "Tell me about it from the beginning."
- "Tell me more about that..."
- "What happened next?"
- "What has been going on from when you first noticed the diarrhea up until now?"
- "What are your thoughts on what might be causing his lameness?"
- "How has Max been doing since our last appointment?"

How questions are asked influences the data-gathering process [20,21]. Eliciting the full range of concerns during the data-gathering portion of the veterinary clinical interview has implications for the quality and outcomes of care, including appointment length, late-arising problems, premature hypothesis generation and testing, diagnostic accuracy, client satisfaction, adherence to recommendations, and patient health. Open-ended questioning encourages the client to tell his or her story and ensures that the client reveals the full spectrum of concerns. Closed-ended questioning limits the field of inquiry and may obstruct the client from revealing his or her full spectrum of concerns; it can also result in decreased accuracy in data collection and increased chances of "hidden concerns" arising at the end of the visit. Use of open-ended questions aids in understanding the client's perspective and promotes client participation, enhancing client satisfaction and client adherence to recommendations [22].

Research findings indicate that veterinarians use primarily closed-ended questioning to gather data [23]. In general, 13 closed-ended questions (range: 0–42 questions) were used per appointment compared with 2 open-ended questions (range: 0–11 questions). In 75 of 300 appointments (25%), veterinarians did not use any open-ended questioning. Although a standard prescription of the number of open-ended questions to ask per clinical interview does not exist, a general recommendation is to use a funnel approach to data gathering [8]. This means beginning the interview with broad, exploratory, open-ended questions and progressing to more specific, direct, closed-ended questions to clarify details.

Reflective Listening

Reflective listening goes hand in hand with open-ended questioning. Reflective listening entails reflecting back in your own words the content or feelings behind the person's message (ie, "It sounds like you are worried that he might be blocked again") [8]. Reflective listening demonstrates your interest in the client and your desire to understand what the client is saying [19]. Reflective listening presents a one-way mirror to the client, allowing the client to see oneself and to know that he or she has been heard. Importantly, reflective listening provides an opportunity for the client to clarify, correct, confirm, or add information, enhancing the accuracy of data gathering. In summary, reflective listening enables you to check whether your own interpretation is correct, ensuring accuracy in the clinical interview and encouraging client input.

Techniques for reflective listening include echoing, paraphrasing, and summarizing. Echoing involves repeating the last few words that a client said (ie, "So, Friskie threw up twice last night") [8]. Paraphrasing is to restate in your own words the content or feelings behind the client's message (ie, "I am glad that you brought him in today. It sounds like you and Friskie had a tough morning") [8]. Summarizing is presenting an explicit summary to the client of the information gathered thus far (ie, "Can I see if I have got this right? Friskie vomited twice last night. He seemed fine up until that point. After dinner, you found Friskie licking off one of the plates, and you are wondering whether he may have eaten something that upset his stomach. Is that right?") [8].

Examples
- "So, you are saying that you're frustrated with his response to treatment."
- "It sounds like this is really distressing for you."

- "You are wondering if this surgery is a wise decision."
- "I hear you saying that you're not sure that relocating is the best idea."
- "I sense that you are feeling overwhelmed with making this decision."

Little research has been conducted specifically investigating the use of reflective listening in clinical interviews. In one study, primary care physicians who used paraphrasing and interpretation were less likely to have a history of malpractice claims [24]. Research findings indicate that reflective listening is an underused tool in veterinary clinical interviews [23]. Approximately 50% of veterinary visits included paraphrasing and interpreting client statements.

Empathy Statements

In a general sense, to be empathetic is to put yourself in someone else's shoes or to see a problem from another person's position [8]. It is important to distinguish empathy from sympathy. Empathy is viewing a situation from the client's perspective, whereas sympathy is feeling pity or concern from outside of the client's position. There is a difference in responding empathetically to someone's predicament internally and actually demonstrating empathy externally toward another person through expression of an empathic statement (ie, "I sense how angry you have been feeling about Max's cancer diagnosis").

There are two tasks in creating an empathetic response [8]. The first is to appreciate another person's predicament or feelings. The second step is to communicate that understanding back to the client in a supportive manner (ie, "I sense how difficult it is for you to talk about this"). Expression of empathy is strengthened when accompanied by empathic nonverbal communication, including facial expressions, proximity, touch, tone of voice, or use of silence.

Examples
- "I can see how hard it is to make this decision."
- "It must have been difficult for you raise this concern with me."
- "It sounds like you did all that you could for Molly."
- "It must have been scary to go through that alone."

Building a relationship is vital to the success of every appointment, and expressing empathy is central to building a relationship [10]. Use of empathic statements validates the client's concerns for his or her pet's health and aids in building trust and rapport, because the client feels as though he or she has been truly heard and accepted [10]. A trusting relationship enables the client to tell his or her story and share concerns, helps to prevent misunderstanding and conflict, and promotes client and physician satisfaction [13,25,26]. Rapport-building behaviors are highly valued by clients. In the KPMG study, pet owners ranked "The veterinarian is kind and gentle" first in importance in choosing a veterinarian [1]. In addition, pet owners ranked veterinarians first in compassion, honesty, and trustworthiness in comparison to other professionals (ie, physician, accountant, chiropractor, lawyer, dentist, teacher, pharmacist). Building a strong veterinarian-client-patient relationship promotes client satisfaction [27–29].

Research findings indicate that empathy statements are underused in veterinary appointments [23]. Veterinarians expressed empathy statements in only 7% of appointments. In the study conducted by Bylund and Makoul [30], 60% (100/168) of the clinical encounters had at least one empathic opportunity, and an overall mean of 2.49 empathic opportunities was identified per clinical encounter. The results of this study indicate that an empathic opportunity exists in the majority of clinical interviews. Results of the Shaw et al study reported that veterinarians expressed empathy in only 7% of veterinary visits. Using the Bylund and Makoul study as a general indication of the number of empathic opportunities in clinical encounters, it appears that veterinarians in the Shaw et al study missed empathic opportunities.

IMPLEMENTATION

The key steps to teaching and learning clinical communication skills are as follows [8]:

1. Delineation of the skills
2. Observation of skill use
3. Self-reflection on videotaped interactions
4. Feedback
5. Opportunities for practice

The focus of the first part of this article is defining and delineating the four core communication skills to enhance clinical outcomes. The next step in skill development is to create opportunities for observation, self-reflection, feedback, and practice within the clinical setting.

Methods for Teaching Communication Skills

Communication is a learned skill and can be taught [8]. Experiential learning techniques have been favored over traditional didactic lectures, and the use of small groups and videotaped or live patients or role-playing actors, together with observation and constructive feedback, has been shown to be far more successful than didactic teaching in terms of skill performance. Teaching methods include self- and peer assessment, provision of descriptive and nonjudgmental positive feedback and constructively phrased negative feedback, offering suggestions for alternative phrasing and behavior, and participant practice. The training program should involve repeated practice with guidance and feedback [31]. This repetitive process reinforces learning efforts and builds skills over time. Communication skills are best taught by providing safe and supportive opportunities to practice [8].

Communication teaching is performance based and, in the academic setting, involves working in small groups with simulated clients, using practice-based scenarios, under the guidance of a communication coach, who provides descriptive and constructive feedback [8]. Simulated clients are professionals, who have been carefully screened, coached, and trained to express the vast range of client interactions that veterinarians experience in practice realistically. Using cases based on real practice situations and interactions with simulated clients creates the opportunity for students to develop communication skills in a safe and supportive environment in preparation for the day they serve clients in the hospital. Videotaping of simulated client interactions provides an opportunity for students to reflect on their performance and to identify areas of strength and areas for further development.

Videotaping

Videotaping is recognized as the gold standard of communication teaching, and self-assessment is an important part of analysis of a clinical interview [8,32,33]. Skill development is enhanced through self-observation and reflection of videotaped interactions. Watching yourself on videotape creates an opportunity to identify what you are doing and how you might enhance your performance. Particular sections of the clinical interview can be revisited to focus on the use of particular skills, and the videotape can be reviewed at later dates to assess skill development over time.

It is important to obtain client consent before videotaping. In the author's experience, clients are willing to consent to videotaping of veterinary visits to enhance veterinarian-client-patient communication. Client consent can be obtained through an oral discussion (see the following example), followed by the signing of a consent form. With the advent of digital technology and the associated reduction in camera size, a tripod-mounted videocamera can be unobtrusively set up in even a small examination room.

Example
"I am working on enhancing my client communication skills and was wondering if it would be okay with you if I videotaped today's visit. If any concerns were to arise during the visit, I will turn off the videocamera at any time. The videotape will only be used for my learning process and will not be shared with anyone else."

Putting It into Practice
Create opportunities for communication skills training in the practice setting using existing resources.

Setting Communication Learning Objectives
The first step in learning a skill is to identify your personal communication learning objectives. Effective learning objectives are SMART (specific, measurable, attainable, realistic, and trackable). For example, a general objective would be to "become a better communicator." A more specific objective would be to "demonstrate use of open-ended inquiry and reflective listening when interviewing clients during the week." It is possible to measure the number of times that you ask open-ended versus closed-ended questions and the number of reflective listening statements you used and to monitor your progress in the use of these skills over time. In addition, you can determine the number of times you would like to use these skills in one clinical interview to ensure that your learning objective is realistic and attainable.

Identifying a Communication Coach

The role of the coach is to empower the learner to achieve performance at a higher level through observation, problem solving, instruction, encouragement, and constructive feedback [8]. The ideal coach has the learner's best interests in mind and fosters a trusting relationship. Choose someone who you think meets these criteria and will best support your learning. Inform your coach of your personal communication learning objectives, and request that your coach observe you conducting clinical interviews. If possible, set aside time immediately after the clinical interview to debrief with your coach and to receive feedback on your performance, and set aside time later in the day to review your videotape while the interaction is still fresh in your mind.

Effective Feedback

The success of the coach-practitioner interaction is dependent on the quality of feedback provided by the coach and the practitioner's receptivity to feedback. Guidelines for effective feedback are listed below [8]:

- Feedback should be descriptive rather than judgmental or evaluative.
- Make feedback specific rather than general.
- Focus feedback on behavior rather than on personality.
- Limit feedback to the amount of information that the recipient can use rather than the amount you want to give.
- Focus on sharing information rather than on giving advice.
- Check out interpretations of feedback
- Be well intentioned, valuing, and supportive.

Videotape Self-Reflection

Watching yourself on videotape can be a challenging and enlightening experience, and using a structure approach may provide helpful guidance. Watch the videotape the first time without taking notes to get past the natural responses of watching yourself on videotape. Watch the videotape a second time taking notes and recording your initial impressions and reactions. Watch the videotape a third time, and focus on the learning objectives you set yourself to achieve. The following guiding questions may be helpful to you in the self-reflection process [34]:

- What strengths in your clinical communication skills did this interaction demonstrate?
- What learning needs did this interaction reveal to you?
- Which one learning need do you wish to address as a priority?
- What actions are you going to take to achieve this?
- How will you know when you have reached your target?

Opportunities for Practice

Given the importance of repetition and reinforcement to skill development [31], create a timeline for objective setting, observation, feedback, and videotape self-reflection at various time periods based on your individual needs. Different client interactions may trigger your interest in re-evaluating your clinical communication skills. It may be a good learning experience to videotape yourself in diverse interactions with clients, including wellness, problem, and emergency appointments; clients of differing genders, ages, and educational and socioeconomic backgrounds; varying species of animals; new clients and long-standing clients; and clients who are easy to converse with and clients whom you find challenging. This process may help you to identify some constructive solutions to communicating with a myriad of clients.

SUMMARY

For 40 years, medical researchers have been studying physician-patient interactions, and the results of these studies have yielded three basic conclusions: physician-patient interactions have an impact on patient health, patient and physician satisfaction, adherence to medical recommendations, and malpractice risk; communication is a core clinical skill and an essential component of clinical competence [8]; and appropriate training programs can significantly change medical practitioners' communication knowledge, skills, and attitudes. Many of these findings are applicable to the practice of veterinary medicine. Although research on veterinarian-client-patient communication is lacking in veterinary medicine, we accept that the trust and rapport that results from a healthy veterinarian-client-patient relationship has the potential to motivate clients to make appointments, show up on time, consent to treatment, follow recommendations, pay their bills on time, and refer other people [35]. The end result is personal and professional success resulting from healthy long-term veterinarian-client-patient interactions. It is clear that a focus on interpersonal interactions in veterinary medicine is essential to the ongoing evolution of the profession.

References

[1] Brown JP, Silverman JD. The current and future market for veterinarians and veterinary medical services in the United States. J Am Vet Med Assoc 1999;215:161–83.

[2] Cron WL, Slocum JV, Goodnight DB, et al. Executive summary of the Brakke management and behavior study. J Am Vet Med Assoc 2000;217:332–8.

[3] Lewis RE, Klausner JS. Nontechnical competencies underlying career success as a veterinarian. J Am Vet Med Assoc 2003;222:1690–6.

[4] American Animal Hospital Association. The path to high quality care: practical tips for improving compliance. Lakewood (CO): American Animal Hospital Association; 2003.

[5] Blackwell MJ. The 2001 Inverson Bell Symposium Keynote Address: beyond philosophical differences: the future training of veterinarians. J Vet Med Educ 2001;28:148–52.

[6] Russell RL. Preparing veterinary students with the interactive skills to effectively work with clients and staff. J Vet Med Educ 1994;21:40–3.

[7] Shaw JR, Adams CL, Bonnett BN. What can veterinarians learn from studies of physician-patient communication about veterinarian-client-patient communication? J Am Vet Med Assoc 2004;224:676–84.

[8] Kurtz SM, Silverman J, Draper J. Teaching and learning communication skills in medicine. Arbingdon (UK): Radcliffe Medical Press; 2005.

[9] Chadderdon LM, King LJ, Lloyd JW. The skills, knowledge, aptitudes and attitudes of successful veterinarians: a summary of presentations to the NCVEI subgroup (Brook Lodge, Augusta, Michigan, December 4–6, 2000). J Vet Med Educ 2001;28:28–30.

[10] Silverman J, Kurtz SA, Draper J. Skills for communicating with patients. Arbingdon (UK): Radcliffe Medical Press; 2005.

[11] Lagoni L, Butler C, Hetts S. The human-animal bond and grief. Philadelphia: WB Saunders; 1994.

[12] Emanuel EJ, Emanuel LJ. Four models of the physician-patient relationship. JAMA 1992;267:2221–6.

[13] Buller MK, Buller DB. Physicians' communication style and patient satisfaction. J Health Soc Behav 1987;28:375–88.

[14] Roter DL. The enduring and evolving nature of the patient-physician relationship. Patient Educ Couns 2000;39:5–15.

[15] Bonvicini K. Bayer Animal Health Communication Project. It goes without saying: non-verbal communication in veterinarian-client relationships. New Haven (CT): Institute for Healthcare Communication; 2004.

[16] Hall JA, Roter DL, Katz NR. Task versus socioemotional behaviors in physicians. Med Care 1987;25:399–412.

[17] Hall JA, Roter DL, Rand CS. Communication of affect between patient and physician. J Health Soc Behav 1981;22:18–30.

[18] Weinberger M, Greene JY, Mamlin JJ. The impact of clinical encounter events on patient and physician satisfaction. Soc Sci Med 1981;15E(Suppl):239–44.

[19] Bonvicini K. Bayer Animal Health Communication Project. Getting the story: understanding client and patient. New Haven (CT): Institute for Healthcare Communication; 2003.

[20] Beckman HB, Frankel RM. The effect of physician behavior on the collection of data. Ann Intern Med 1984;101:692–6.

[21] Marvel MK, Epstein RM, Flowers K, et al. Soliciting the patient's agenda, have we improved? JAMA 1999;281:283–7.

[22] Roter DL, Hall JA. Physicians' interviewing styles and medical information obtained from patients. J Gen Intern Med 1987;2:325–9.

[23] Shaw JR, Adams CL, Bonnett BN, et al. A description of veterinarian-client-patient communication using the Roter Method of Interaction Analysis. J Am Vet Med Assoc 2004;225: 222–9.

[24] Levinson W, Roter DL, Mullooly JP, et al. Physician-patient communication: the relationship with malpractice claims among primary care physicians and surgeons. JAMA 1997;277: 553–9.

[25] Bertakis KD, Roter DL, Putnam SM. The relationship of physician medical interview style to patient satisfaction. J Fam Pract 1991;32:175–81.

[26] Levinson W, Stiles WB, Inui TS, et al. Physician frustration in communicating with patients. Med Care 1993;31:285–95.

[27] Antelyes J. Client hopes, client expectations. J Am Vet Med Assoc 1990;197:1596–7.

[28] Antelyes J. Difficult clients in the next decade. J Am Vet Med Assoc 1991;198:550–2.

[29] Case DB. Survey of expectations among clients of three small animal clinics. J Am Vet Med Assoc 1988;192:498–502.

[30] Bylund CL, Makoul G. Empathic communication and gender in the physician-patient encounter. Patient Educ Couns 2002;48:207–16.

[31] Hulsman RL, Ros WJG, Winnubst JAM, et al. Teaching clinically experienced physicians communication skills: a review of evaluation studies. Med Educ 1999;33:655–68.

[32] Beckman HB, Frankel RM. The use of videotape in internal medicine training. J Gen Intern Med 1994;9:517–21.

[33] Ram P, Grol R, Rethans JJ, et al. Assessment of general practitioners by video observation of communicative and medical performance in daily practice: issues of validity, reliability and feasibility. Med Educ 1999;33:447–54.

[34] Pee B, Woodman T, Fry H, et al. Appraising and assessing reflection in students' writing on a structured worksheet. Med Educ 2002;36:575–85.

[35] Antelyes J. Client husbandry. J Am Vet Med Assoc 1988;192:166–8.

Vet Clin Small Anim 36 (2006) 397–409

VETERINARY CLINICS
SMALL ANIMAL PRACTICE

Move Your Practice to New Heights with Down-To-Earth Hiring Techniques

Bonita S. Voiland, MS*

Cornell University Hospital for Animals, College of Veterinary Medicine,
Box 20, Ithaca, NY 14853, USA

THE VIEW FROM THE TARMAC

Reflecting on the state of veterinary medicine using a pundit's view from 50,000 feet can be enlightening, but to assure everyday success, veterinary practice owners need to have their feet firmly on the tarmac.

Consider a sampling of decisions your employees make daily: Should I tell this client there are no appointments open today, so I can knock off early? Should I mop the kennel floor even though it doesn't look dirty? Should this client be given a break on the bill even though the practice will not recoup the expense of the care provided?

None of those single decisions will make or break a practice. Taken together, however, the sum of employees' actions influences everything from the reputation of each individual who works in the practice to how much money the practice will net this year. You cannot be at the practice 24/7, monitoring every decision made by every employee. What's a practice owner to do?

IT'S ABOUT THE 'FIT'—BUT THE FIT TO WHAT?

This article is about recruiting and hiring the right people to work in your practice so you do not have to monitor every decision. If you agree that your practice cannot thrive without good employees, then hiring good people becomes one of the most important aspects of practice management.

Hiring the right people starts with knowing what kind of culture you want in your practice, just as you must know what kinds of cases you want to treat. Your own leadership style and your employees' attitudes about work are important facilitators to achieving practice goals, but they can also be formidable obstacles unless there is a congruence and consistency to support your practice's work environment—its culture—according to academic researchers and experienced practitioners [1].

*Correspondence. Box 20, Veterinary Medical Center, Ithaca, NY 14853. *E-mail address:* bsv2@cornell.edu

0195-5616/06/$ – see front matter
doi:10.1016/j.cvsm.2005.10.006

Culture is essential to consider because it affects teamwork and impacts every employee's ability to get the job done. Researchers also have suggested that a practice's culture can provide a competitive edge [2,3]. Most academics have settled on a definition of culture as "a practical pattern of beliefs and expectations that are more or less shared by the organization's members. These beliefs and expectations produce norms that can powerfully shape the employees' behavior" [2]. In practical terms, your practice's culture is a system of values and behavioral norms shared by you and your employees.

Whether you are a practice owner or you are looking for your first job, if you have not reflected on the kind of environment you want to work in, do so. Start by assessing whether the structures of individual jobs, the formal and informal information flow within the practice, and the work environment are consistent with the direction in which you want the business to head. Inconsistencies in any of these areas can be the root causes of performance problems at every level of the practice and can result in lost reputation, lost business, and lost net revenue.

A culture that values participatory teamwork may hold frequent staff meetings that include every employee and encourage everyone's input, host training sessions for all employees in teamwork and communication skills, and base pay increases for hourly employees on overall team performance as well as on the employee's ability to demonstrate initiative and flexibility within the context of the team. In such a culture, a new-to-the-practice office manager who announces a change in office hours without first obtaining input and feedback from the rest of the staff could expect employee resistance based on the violation of the cultural norm.

A culture that is doctor-centered may exclude non-veterinarians from staff meetings, limit training opportunities to veterinarians only, and limit incentive-based salary increases to the veterinarian staff. A technician who believes in the value of continuously improving technical skills would unlikely stay at the practice if he or she finds another practice that pays for technical continuing education sessions or makes time available for the technician to seek advanced certification or be involved in state professional associations.

Practically, culture creates a self-monitoring behavioral control system within an organization: "Control is the knowledge that someone who knows and cares is paying close attention to what we do and can tell us when deviations are occurring" [4]. The control does not have to be heavy handed to be effective. For example, a few years ago, when the head of a major airline was worried about his airline's on-time record, he personally requested a daily report of the on-time status of all flights. Within 2 years, on-time performance rose from 83% to 97% [5]. When a practice manager walks through the kennels several times every day, noticing and sincerely complimenting the staff on the cleanliness and the way in which the staff interacts with the animals, that also is a control mechanism that communicates to the staff that those functions are important to the people who do the hiring and who have input on promotions and raises.

Asking for a daily report or walking through the kennels several times a day is one matter. What about situations that are not routine or predictable? The situations that are most challenging—and during which the practice is at greatest risk—are those that cannot be scripted and that require creativity, an immediate judgment call, and flexibility on the part of the decision maker. In these situations a practice's employees must rely on their own value system and their understanding of what they are expected to resolve and will be rewarded for resolving. If within the practice a culture has developed in which employees agree on and mutually enforce certain standards of behavior, then the practice's culture functions as a social control system to keep decision-making on track, consistent with the practice's values.

These norms form "expectations about what constitute appropriate or inappropriate attitudes and behaviors, socially created standards that help us interpret and evaluate events" [4]. Norms can be important (eg, those related to how flexible work schedules are or how conflict is dealt with) or less important (eg, the color of the scrubs the techs wear). Whether important or not, norms can help or hinder the attainment of a particular strategy within the practice. For instance, routinely singling out an individual to receive an employee-of-the-month honor may be counterproductive if the goal is to foster an overall team environment. Likewise some poorly constructed financial incentive plans for entry-level associates have fostered competitiveness at the overall expense of turnover and the practice's bottom line.

Likewise, there will be problems if there are differences between the values and the norms held by the practice owner and the other employees of the practice. O'Reilly [4] defines the former as a reflection of the way the owner wants things to be, whereas the latter reflect how things actually are. O'Reilly also differentiates between how firmly norms are held by employees by using of a matrix with one axis representing high or low intensity (the amount of approval or disapproval attached to each expectation) and the other axis representing high- or low consensus (the consistency with which the norm is held). An example of a norm with high consensus but low intensity, which O'Reilly terms "a vacuous belief," may exist around expectations of how long clients should wait before being seen in an examination room: everyone may understand that the practice owner wants clients to be greeted in an examination room by a veterinary technician within 5 minutes of the scheduled time of the appointment, but when the practice owner is not monitoring performance, clients routinely languish without explanation in the reception area for 20 or 30 or minutes or longer. The opposite panel in O'Reilly's matrix would house an example of low consensus but high intensity, such as a situation in which a practice's associate prescribes hourly kennel monitoring by after-hours staff, but the kennel staff surf the Internet on the office computer instead of actually checking on the animals.

All this discussion may ring true, but how does a practice owner create commitment among staff to norms that assure a self-monitoring culture consistent with the owner's vision? From a prospective job applicant's perspective, how does the applicant determine whether a practice's culture will foster a sense of job involvement and loyalty?

Both potential employer and potential employee are seeking congruence, which starts with understanding how commitment is created [6]. O'Reilly and Chatman [7] identified three stages of commitment: compliance, identification, and internalization. Compliance is the most fragile stage of commitment. Compliance occurs as an exchange, for instance, when an applicant accepts the norm of being on time for work in exchange for getting the desired objective, that is, obtaining a job. "Of course I will be here on time every day," the applicant for a kennel job may state in an interview. An employee whose norms of acceptable work behavior had not been formed previously would take cues from role models and the culture within the practice to determine if being on time is important. In this case, the employee may not identify that being on time is valued in this practice if the practice manager often shows up 15 minutes late for work or associates are habitually late for staff meetings. If on-time expectations have been stated, if there are consequences to being late, and if all staff are consistently on time, the employee will learn the on-time norm more quickly. When employment represents something attractive to the person (the job itself is intrinsically rewarding to the individual, it represents a means of gaining experience for a veterinary school application, or the wages themselves are important), the employee is more likely to move from compliance to identification with the practice's normative behaviors.

The highest level of commitment is internalization, in which the employee finds the practice's values and norms to be intrinsically rewarding and congruent with personal values. Internalized norms provide powerful self-monitoring behavior, regardless of the presence of external monitors, such as the presence of the practice owner in the previous example.

WE ARE HIRING—WHAT NOW?

Researchers have studied in depth the individual–organization fit (ie, how well a person's values and norms mesh with those of an organization's culture) and how to identify a potential employee's fit within a particular organization. The veterinary profession has followed suit [8]. The National Commission on Veterinary Economic Issues obtained funding to identify and hone the list of skills, knowledge, aptitudes, and abilities (SKAs) necessary for veterinary students to be successful upon graduation. The same type of analysis can be extended to all positions within a practice to assure the there is good congruence between potential employees' SKAs and the jobs they will be performing in the practice. To hire employees who are capable of internalizing your practice's norms, you need to look specifically at the job for which you are recruiting. Make sure a current, written job description provides adequate detail about the job. The job description should be more than a checklist of duties and responsibilities, however. Like many large organizations, Cornell University's Office of Human Resources has created "Staff Skills for Success," descriptions of which are incorporated into every university job description. The document describes the university's expectations of every employee in the areas of communication, teamwork, flexibility, initiative, and more. Those skill expectations are used to start the process of setting norms and expectations while interviewing and orienting new staff, and later the standards are considered as part of annual performance evaluations, to determine continuing education and training plans, and to establish pay raises [9].

After you have a good job description, give some careful thought to the organizational levers for shaping culture, obtaining good individual–organization fit, and achieving more than compliance with work rules.

Recruitment, Selection, and Hiring

Matters to consider in recruiting, selecting, and hiring staff are

- Who does my practice attract? Are these the people we want to attract? How are we communicating what we are looking for?
- Who do we select? Do these people typically work out, or do they tend to leave in relatively short order?

Orientation, Training, and Socialization

In orientation, training, and socialization of new employees, consider

- Are our values and mission written?
- Can every person in the practice do a decent job of articulating the practice's mission and values?

If you answer "no" to any question, search "writing a mission statement" on the Web to find excellent Web sites that will provide guidance. Then take an hour and discuss with the entire staff (kennel staff, receptionists, technicians, veterinarians—everyone) why they think you are in the business you are in and how they think the practice should be delivering service. Then make an attempt to write down the consensus. Discuss your draft with the staff again. The practice owner has the final say, but the mission statement will be a lot more than a "vacuous belief" if everyone has input and a chance to really think about it. Matters to discuss and incorporate in the mission statement include

- What values does your practice hold? How are the values of the practice communicated to new employees? Do you talk about them frequently? Do they matter?
- Are there written rules, polices, procedures? How and when are they given to new employees? Who/what kind of person passes along the unwritten "rules" to new employees?
- How does the practice really run? To what extent are the values and norms of the practice's informal organization structure consistent with those of the formal organization?

Role Models

In considering role models, think about

- Who/what kinds of people are formal leaders of the practice?
- Who/what kinds of people are the informal leaders of the practice?

- To what extent do norms, values, and internal working relationships help get tasks accomplished?

Rewards and Recognition

Address the following questions when thinking about rewards and recognition:

- Are there regular performance reviews? Are there other opportunities to regularly talk about career goals or how things are going on the job?
- Is input welcome from everyone? Is input acted upon?
- Are there regular pay increases? Is pay tied to individual or team performance?
- Who/what kind of person is selected to be rewarded financially or by promotion?
- Who/what kind of person leaves your practice? After how long? Is turnover in certain job categories desirable?
- Is task performance helped or hindered by the way this practice is structured formally and informally? What are the barriers that prevent someone from doing an outstanding job? Can those barriers be removed?
- Is this particular job designed to be inherently rewarding? If not, can duties be added or shuffled to make it more than it currently is?

The Right Person the First Time: Recruitment, Selection, and Hiring

Public relations professionals define an organization's identity as the mission and values that the people running the organization want the company to be known for, whereas image is what various constituencies perceive to be the reality about the organization's mission and values. An organization's image influences how attractive the company is to potential job applicants and how likely job seekers are to apply for a position within that organization [10]. Research confirms that visibility, social networks, and traditional recruitment practices are positively related to job seekers' initial organizational images [11]. Unlike large corporations, veterinary practices do not have the means to purchase image advertising or otherwise influence the general public's image on a grand scale. Practices can, however, take full advantage of public relations efforts, social networks, and traditional recruitment practices to make the most of their recruitment efforts. Practice personnel who participate in community public service efforts such as charity runs or community clean-up efforts both help their community and assist in recruiting people who like to help their communities, especially if staff members are wearing T-shirts or other apparel that readily identifies the practice while they participate in these events.

Most North American schools of veterinary medicine have formal and informal career-placement activities open to both alumni and non-alumni. Often overlooked, however, are the opportunities that exist at schools of veterinary technology to connect your practice with recent graduates and alumni who are using the school's networking system to seek jobs. If your area is chronically short of qualified veterinary technicians, consider offering paid or unpaid internships to get to know veterinary technicians-in-training. The authors' hospital has had excellent success with an externship program that offers veterinary technology students the opportunity to explore specialty practice and to hone basic skills in a structured environment, and it has given the hospital staff the chance to evaluate the skills and fit of participants for potential future employment.

These efforts have a sound basis in research. Familiarity with a potential employer and with the employer's reputation and image has significant and independent direct effects on application behaviors. Research suggests that employers can recruit more successfully if they use strategies that match the extent to which their practice is known by potential applicants [12]. General familiarity with a potential employer and the employer's reputation are essential factors that increase job seekers' motivation to apply for jobs or to seek out additional information. A company's brand visibility (image) is the first source that job seekers may draw upon to develop these opinions [13,14]. In the absence of a strong and visible image among potential job applicants, a practice must find alternative ways to create initial positive familiarity in the minds of job seekers. Low-information practices such as banner advertisements, recruiting posters, and sponsorship of campus or community events also affect job seekers' attitudes toward a practice by exposing them to positive signals about the practice.

Such activities do not seem to have significant effects on job seekers in companies that have high brand visibility (eg, veterinary teaching hospitals), because these low-information activities provide information that is essentially redundant to the organization's known image. For companies that are already generally familiar to applicants, high-information recruitment practices such as detailed recruitment advertisements and brochures and employee (alumni, intern) endorsements positively influence job seekers to apply or seek more information [14].

There are similar choices to make in advertising prose. Other research has shown that employers who wish to attract fewer but more qualified individuals should write advertisements with job descriptions relating to the work itself plus specific information related to the abilities required to do the job. This information gives the more unqualified candidates the opportunity to screen themselves out because they lack a match with the job. If the purpose of the advertisement is to attract as many qualified applicants as possible (eg, if you are seeking technicians who have requisite base skills but whom you intend to train to a specialty job function), an advertisement that describes information relating to the job and the work itself will bring more applicants from which to choose [15].

Visibility, social networks, and recruitment practices are positively related to job seekers' initial images of organizations. Because there is a positive correlation with initial images and the job seekers' exposure to job postings, recruitment brochures, and Websites for organizations previously unknown to them [11], practices would be wise to invest in professional design and copywriting to help to create materials that cut through ambient media clutter.

They're Here! Now What?

Once there is a good pool of applicants, what is next? If picking the right people to work in your practice was an easy task, all you would have to do is get a bunch of smart people in a room, and great things would happen. But the process does not work like that. In fact, recent research by Casciaro and Lobo [16] shows when employees need help in getting a job done, they gravitate toward individuals who are team players rather than those who may have more task-specific knowledge but who are known to be difficult to work with. Employees' choices with whom they collaborate validate that job knowledge is only one dimension of the necessary skill set. In fact, a person's means of communication and collegially are actually more important than task competence if a negative personality inhibits the team from accessing that person's knowledge base. An employee whom researchers Casciaro and Lobo term a "competent jerk" may never have the chance to benefit the practice as a whole, because other employees in the practice will avoid working with that individual.

It is no surprise that researchers found that interviewers are more likely to offer jobs to those they think fit well with their organizations, and that applicants will be attracted to and prefer employment with organizations with which they feel a greater fit [17]. Just how well both applicants and employers assess that fit during the recruitment and interviewing process is the key to successful hiring. Such assessment is no simple matter. In a health care setting such as a veterinary practice, technical skill often is emphasized over all other skills. That emphasis can lead to hiring the "competent jerk," at a price your practice staff—and you—will have to pay.

Like the sports equivalent, a work team is only as good as its weakest member. To maximize the team's performance, use the interview process to identify the person who has the potential to perform at peak levels technically and interpersonally within your practice. Give the interview process your attention and your time to get it right.

Sort through the applications
- Always require a cover letter in addition to a resume or a standard fill-in-the-blank application form for any position. Screen the documents for how well, how neatly, and how thoughtfully they are prepared. How a person organizes his or her thoughts tells you something about how that person might organize the workday or how well the person can communicate verbally.
- Screen the resume again for qualifications and experience.
- Sort the applications into three piles. In pile A place resumes of qualified applicants whose presentation of information you like. These are persons you definitely will interview. In pile B place resumes for persons who are not as well qualified or whose presentation was not as thoughtful as those in the A group. You will consider these persons for an interview. In pile C place resumes that are out of the running. Unless you made a mistake the first time through the applications, do not consider anyone in the C group for the job, even if you have to re-advertise and beat the bushes for additional applicants. If you hire from group C, you are asking for a misfit.

Pre-screen on the telephone
- Contact the candidate and set up a mutually convenient time to have an initial phone conversation.
- Listen well to the person's answers to your questions; make notes. This interview can save you time in the long run and eliminate the temptation to make a judgment based on visual cues and first (visual) impressions. Herb Greenberg, CEO of Caliper, a human-resource consulting firm that has evaluated more than 2 million job candidates and employees for its clients, said in a 2005 interview, "Most people depend too much on their sight … The key to hiring and managing people is to find out what drives them. One of the most important questions to ask is 'Why?' … People can work on their smile … but voices are genuine. You can tell if the person is comfortable with you (or) if there's no reaching out in their voice. When someone's voice is flat or quiet … that can be a warning flag … You can have all the talent in the world and not be able to make use of those strengths if you lack the character and determination and enthusiasm" [18].

Invite the most promising applicants for a face-to-face interview
The authors consider the interview an opportunity to sell their practice to the individual as well as to ascertain whether the person will make an appropriate member of their team. They want everyone who is interviewed at their hospital to feel respected and positive about the experience, whether or not the person is hired, because even applicants who are not hired can be ambassadors if the interviewers do a good job during the interview.

- The authors require applicants to spend at least a half-day with them.
- Written information about the job is mailed in advance, including the interview schedule that includes the names and titles of the people with whom they will meet; the job description including Staff Skills for Success; the hospital mission statement and, if the position is a technical position, the values statement written by the technicians; and Website addresses, maps, and information about housing, recreation, and schools obtained from the local Chamber of Commerce.
- When the interview day arrives, after a welcome and initial talk with the hiring supervisor, every applicant is given a tour of the hospital. Then for a minimum of 2 hours the applicant shadows one or two high-performing staff members who can show him or her what the job is like. This procedure gives the applicant time to see what is really expected and to ask questions in a more relaxed atmosphere, and it gives the authors the chance to assess the applicant.
- The applicant and staff share a light lunch in the break room so more team members can interact with the applicant.
- After shadowing and lunch, there is second conversation with the hiring supervisor to answer any final questions and get the applicant's impressions of the day and the job.
- The authors ask each applicant to think about the experience and call in the next day or two to say whether he or she is still interested in the job. The authors explain where they are in the hiring process and when they will be making the decision about the finalists for the position.

Take another look; then let the right person make the hiring decision

After every applicant's visit, the hiring supervisor gets written input from everyone who interacted with the individual. These are the questions:

- Please comment on this person's team skills. What skills does this person have to qualify him or her for this position? Do you have any concerns about this person's ability to actively and ably participate as a member of a diverse team of people? What leadership skills does this person exhibit?
- Please comment on this person's technical skills relative to the demands of this position.
- Do you think this person would be successful in this position and contribute to the overall purpose of the service to which they are applying and the mission of the hospital? Why or why not?

The hiring supervisor then chooses one or two finalists who are invited back to meet for half an hour with the hospital director and practice manager and for one more meeting with the hiring supervisor (if that person is not the director or practice manager). This visit gives another chance to see the applicant and assess the fit with the organization.

The hiring supervisor makes the decision and a verbal job offer.

The verbal job offer is followed up in writing to cement the arrangement.

This process may seem lengthy, but the authors find that it is a good investment of their time compared with the time and stress involved in making wrong hiring decisions.

Assessing congruence: asking the right questions

If you interview an applicant over the telephone and then in person once or twice, you have plenty of time to ask lots of good questions. It is imperative to listen carefully and make brief notes of the applicant's responses. Resist talking too much! The authors' staff often request guidance on the kinds of questions to ask to get a real understanding of how well a person might do in that practice. The authors have compiled a list that they give staff members who will be meeting the candidates and ask them to choose three to four questions that they will consistently ask every candidate. Some suggested questions are given in Box 1.

YOU'RE HIRED! NOW WHAT?

Go back to the process an individual goes through to establish commitment: compliance, identification, and internalization. If you hired well, a new employee will bring a good deal of commitment to the job and the practice. It is important to be sure you are doing everything possible to develop and maintain that commitment at the highest level. Because the practice is only as good as the weakest member of the team, giving attention to the orientation process will move the individual from weakest team member to a fully contributing team member quickly. Everyone in the authors' practice wears an identification badge, and new recruits are no exception. But they also wear a second badge that says, "I'm new here!" to signal to clients and the large staff that this person is in the learning phase.

Box 1: Suggested interview questions

1. To assess if the candidate has the skills, knowledge and abilities
   - What are the three main duties in the job you now have?
   - What special skills or knowledge do you need for those duties?
   - What kinds of decisions do you make and how do you make them?
   - What is the most important thing you have done in your present position?

2. To assess the fit between the individual's aspirations and the practice's mission and values
   - Why do you want to work here?
   - Have you worked with a team like the one you would work with here? Tell about that experience, or what did you like or dislike about the previous experience?
   - When you start a new job, what do you do to help yourself understand the job and the people better? What would you expect from us to help you transition into the job here?
   - What can you tell about your accomplishments in your current job?
   - What will your current employer say about your work performance? Did you have any problems in your current position? How did you handle them? [19]
   - What animals do you have? As an animal owner, what was your best experience at a veterinarian's office? What was the worst? [19]

3. To assess the applicant's needs or desires
   - What do you think you would do for our practice that someone else would not?
   - What kinds of rewards satisfy you most, and how does getting them affect your work?
   - If hired here, how long do you see yourself in this particular job?
   - What do you want to be doing in 5 years?
   - What was the last meaningful continuing education training you attended? What made it so helpful?

4. To assess how the applicant handles conflict
   - Ask for an example of a situation in which the applicant disagreed with a co-worker and how the situation was resolved. Was the result satisfactory?
   - Ask how the applicant handled a disagreement with a supervisor and how it was resolved. Was the result satisfactory?
   - If the applicant has supervised staff, ask how a disagreement with a staff member was handled and resolved. Was the result satisfactory?

The authors' practice is at a large university hospital, and their goal is to make the transition into their practice comfortable and supportive so that long-term success is more assured. Each team leader has a checklist of skills, equipment, and procedures that are assigned to the new employee each week. Initially, the new employee meets weekly with the team leader to discuss progress on these and the Staff Skills for Success. The orientation process is a team responsibility: the new employee is responsible for letting the team leader know what skills he or she wants more practice on, and the team leader and other team members provide feedback on their perceptions of progress. The team leader arranges for dry labs, wet labs, or other activities to assist the new employee make the transition to the sometimes overwhelming practice. At a university hospital devoted to teaching, learning is seen as a career-long progress, so the formal orientation lays the groundwork for ongoing education and training.

From the Ground up: a Firm Foundation Matters
Like preparing for intricate surgery, successful staffing requires preparation, mastery of the subject matter, and skill. The employees who work in veterinary practices form the basis of the business and reflect the owners' own values. Giving attention to what you want your practice to be, whom you want working with you, and how the environment keeps the staff productive matters. Identifying the right culture, hiring people who find congruence with the practice's culture, and consistently applying these principles will help your practice soar to new heights.

Acknowledgment
The author thanks Christopher Collins, PhD, of Cornell University's School of Industrial and Labor Relations, for his guidance in the research of this topic and preparation of this article.

References
[1] Tushman ML, O'Reilly CA III. Winning through innovation: a practical guide to leading organizational change and renewal. Cambridge (MA): Harvard Business School Press; 2002.

[2] Schwartz H, Davis S. Matching corporate culture and business strategy. Organ Dyn 1981;30–48.

[3] Barney J. Organizational culture: can it be a source of sustained competitive advantage? Acad Manage Rev 1986;10:656–65.

[4] O'Reilly C. Managing organization culture: corporations, culture, and commitment: motivation and social control in organizations. Calif Manage Rev 1989;31(4):285–303.

[5] Carlzon J. Moments of truth. Cambridge (MA): Ballinger; 1987.

[6] Mowday R, Porter L, Steers R. Organizational linkages: the psychology of commitment, absenteeism, and turnover. New York: Academic Press; 1982.

[7] O'Reilly C, Chatman J. Organizational commitment and psychological attachment; the effects of compliance, identification and internalization on prosocial behavior. J Appl Psychol 1986;11:285–503.

[8] Greenfield CL, Johnson AL, Schaeffer DJ. Influence of demographic variables on the frequency of use of various procedures, skills, and areas of knowledge among veterinarians in private small-animal practice and proficiency expected of new veterinary school graduates. J Am Vet Med Assoc 2005;226(1):38–48.

[9] Staff skills for success. Cornell University Office of Human Resources, revised 2002, copyright 2005: Available at http://www.ohr.cornell.edu/working/staffPerformanceLearning/skillsSuccess/SFSOverviewChart.doc and http://www.ohr.cornell.edu/working/staffPerformanceLearning/skillsSuccess/skillsSuccessFramework.html. Accessed November 28, 2005.

[10] Gatewood RD, Gowan MA, Lautenschlager GJ. Corporate image, recruitment image, and initial job choice. Acad Manage J 1993;36:414–27.

[11] Collins C, Stevens CK. Initial organizational images and recruitment: a within-subjects investigation of the factors affecting job choices. Presented at the 24th Annual Conference of the Society for Industrial/Organizational Psychology. Atlanta, Georgia, May 1999.

[12] Collins CJ. The interactive effects of recruitment practices and corporate brand visibility on employer knowledge and application behaviors. Ithaca (NY): Cornell University School of Industrial and Labor Relations; 2005.

[13] Cable DM, Turban DB. The value of organizational reputation in the recruitment context: a brand-equity perspective. J Appl Soc Psychol 2003;33:2244–66.

[14] Collins CJ, Han J. Exploring applicant pool quantity and quality: the effects of early recruitment practice strategies, corporate advertising, and firm reputation. Personnel Psychology 2004;57:685–717.

[15] Mason NA, Belt JA. Effectiveness of specificity in recruitment advertising. Journal of Management 1986;12(3):425–32.

[16] Casciaro T, Lobo MS. Competent jerks, lovable fools, and the formation of social networks. Harv Bus Rev 2005;83(6):92–100.

[17] Cable DM, Judge TA. Interviewers' perceptions of person-organization fit and organizational selection decisions. J Appl Psychol 1997;82:546–61.

[18] Greenberg H. Herb Greenberg on interviewing: knowing what to listen for. Harv Bus Rev 2005;83(6):25.

[19] Snyder G. Hiring is the first step. DVM Newsmagazine 2005. Available at: http://www.dvmnews.com/dvm/article/articleDetail.jsp?id=152677.

Vet Clin Small Anim 36 (2006) 411–418

VETERINARY CLINICS
SMALL ANIMAL PRACTICE

Small Animal Practice: Billing, Third-party Payment Options, and Pet Health Insurance

Louise Dunn

Snowgoose Veterinary Management Consulting, 12 Snow Goose Cove, Greensboro, NC 27455, USA

I f there was ever any doubt about pets' status in families or about pet owners' willingness to offer top-notch veterinary care to their pets, just consider the statistics. According to a 2004 report from the American Pet Products Manufacturers Association, pet owners in the United States spend about $16.4 billion on veterinary services [1]. Each year, technological advances give veterinarians the ability to detect and treat more complicated medical cases. Along with advances come rising veterinary costs, to the tune of 7% each year [2]. In 2000, the group reported that surgical veterinary visits accounted for one third to three fourths of pet care expenses. The 2000 survey also found the average income of American pet owners at that time was $36,000, and that 49% earned $35,000 or less [3].

Consider these medical facts: not factoring common breed problems, such as diabetes or hip dysplasia, the Texas A&M College of Veterinary Medicine reports that dogs are 35 times more likely than humans to develop skin cancer, four times more likely to develop a breast tumor, and eight times more likely to suffer from bone cancer [4].

Now consider this financial reality: roughly one of three pet owners say they would make the painful decision to euthanize a pet if medical expenses fall in the $500 to $1000 range [5]. By today's standards, that figure barely covers emergency examination, blood work, radiographs, and surgery fees for a one-time crisis.

Same-day payment for services rendered is not always feasible for financially strapped clients facing several thousand dollars in pet medical bills. Pet health insurance and credit options, made more cost effective through computerized billing or third-party providers, let them accept that much-wanted optimal veterinary care. Are alternative payment options a smart business decision for you and your practice?

E-mail address: snogoose@infionline.net

0195-5616/06/$ – see front matter
doi:10.1016/j.cvsm.2005.10.005

THIRD-PARTY PAYMENT OPTIONS

The National Collection Agency Association reports that for every 30 days a bill goes unpaid, the chance of a business owner seeing any money decreases by 20%. A July 2004 study commissioned by the National Commission of Veterinary Economic Issues (NCVEI) found that NCVEI hospitals with third-party financing had 58% fewer accounts receivable and 22% more revenue [6]. Smart business owners would agree those figures are compelling. Rates and terms vary by company. Practice owners also pay an initial enrollment set-up fee.

CareCredit is a division of GE Consumer Finance. Like many finance companies, CareCredit keeps a percentage of the charge amount, similar to Visa, MasterCard, and other credit card companies. This third-party finance company pays veterinarians the full bill, and clients pay back CareCredit over an agreed period of time. Approved clients can choose from no-interest plans that last 3, 6, or 12 months. Clients in tighter financial straits or with much higher medical bills can choose a low-interest plan for 2, 3, or 4 years.

To initiate the program in a veterinary practice, a CareCredit representative comes on site to set up the terminal, which is similar to a credit card terminal with a keypad. Hospital team members can complete the training session—typically within 1 to 2 hours, on site or even over the telephone—to learn how to manage transactions and applications. All applications take place over the telephone, with approval notification usually granted within a few minutes. The benefits to the practice of using CareCredit include

> Minimal or no treatment negotiation. Doctors can present the treatment course without prejudging clients' ability to pay.
> Minimal or no accounts receivable. CareCredit representatives say practices receive payment within 2 days.
> Ability to offer optimal treatment from the start. There is no need to compromise treatment recommendations while you try to gauge a client's ability to pay.
> Lack of exposure to default. CareCredit assumes full responsibility to collect. If, however, a pet owner for some reason disputes a charge, the company will contact the practice. The practice owner has 30 days to respond. The pet owner must prove that fraud occurred. CareCredit does not judge the quality of veterinary care or services that have been rendered. CareCredit representatives note that these instances are rare, and the pet owner usually agrees to pay the original charges and terms, or an alternate payment arrangement is made. Very rarely, they say, does CareCredit collect money back from the practice.

There is more good news: CareCredit says it will not tag a practice as high-risk and subject it to higher premiums. Like all credit cards, however, CareCredit does have a no-payment default rate for cardholders. It is wise, then, if you use a third-party finance company, to discuss all plan options with clients thoroughly so that they can comfortably make payments on time and in full.

In the fall of 2004, Brakke Consulting Inc. conducted a random-sample survey among 500 pet owners who used CareCredit. It found that [7]

- Seventy-nine percent agreed CareCredit influenced their decision about their pet's treatment.
- Twenty-eight percent of clients surveyed said that, without CareCredit, they would have asked the veterinarian to come up with a less expensive treatment.
- Nineteen percent would have delayed treating their pets.
- Almost 25% of the clients surveyed indicated that they spent more on their pets' veterinary care since obtaining a CareCredit account.

The study showed that clients of veterinary clinics offering CareCredit perceived that the practice was looking out for their best interests, and pet owners believed that they were receiving good value. It also found veterinary clients who finance medical procedures are more likely to follow their veterinarian's recommendations for treatment, are more likely to return to the clinic for additional services, and are more likely to recommend the practice to friends and family.

Contracting with a third-party financier may seem like an obvious step, but before enrolling it is important to study all the options. CareCredit representatives say their plans work best in practices with two, three, or more doctors and in those that focus on surgical or specialty services. Smaller clinics with only one practitioner on staff that tend to focus on spays, neuters, and general wellness care may need alternative payment plans.

Pet Health Insurance

The veterinary profession remains divided on the merits of pet health insurance. The less savory aspects of human managed health care often leave a nasty after taste in the mouths of many veterinarians. Common human health insurance problems include

- Compensation through capitation
- Reduced fee schedules to fit predetermined rates
- Nonmedical personnel deciding what procedures are covered
- Preauthorization battles and paperwork overload

Veterinarians justifiably hesitate to venture down a path where they might have to deal with these troublesome issues. Many also assume pet owners will consider insurance wasted money. The proponents of insurance say this attitude is unwarranted.

"We need to get away from the mentality that insurance is a financial investment and clients can get money back from it," says Dr. James Nave, past president of the American Veterinary Medical Association. "Insurance is protection against disaster." Nothing more.

The general public may not fully understand the difference between managed care and indemnity insurance—two very different things. It would be wise for veterinary medicine to follow human dentists' lead. Dentists rejected managed care and embraced indemnity insurance. According to the Compliance in Companion Animal Practices Study conducted by the American Animal Hospital Association (AAHA), compliance was not a great concern for human dentists. Dental insurance plans now cover an estimated 145 million people in the United States, or approximately 50% of the total population [8]. Dental insurance plans are largely prepaid plans that cover wellness procedures, providing an incentive for a large number of people to obtain the routine care recommended by the profession.

In the United Kingdom, 17% of dog owners and 11% of cat owners have health insurance for emergencies [9]. In Sweden, nearly every other pet is insured. In the United States, less than 0.5% of pets are covered by pet health insurance [5].

Iinsurance is much higher for pedigree pets than for mixed breeds and much higher for dogs than for cats.

Most owners are surprised to learn pet health insurance has been around for decades, but consumer awareness is changing. According to Packaged Facts [10], pet health insurance companies reported a 342% growth between 1999 and 2003. Premiums doubled between 2002 and 2003 alone. Studies of clients who have pet insurance in the United Kingdom find [11]

- Insured pets see veterinarians 30% more often than uninsured pets.
- Clients who have insured pets spend 42% more on average.
- Clients who have insured pets spend 51% more on core services.
- Clients who have insured pets spend 33% more on ancillary services.
- Insured pets are seen an average of 2.6 times a year, compared with an average of twice a year for uninsured pets.

One question remains foremost in the minds of veterinarians and patients everywhere: is the insurance worth the cost? In most cases, pet health insurance is an indemnity contract between the provider and pet owner. One of the most significant but often unmentioned benefits of pet insurance is that, in addition to providing peace of mind and protection against the possibility of experiencing an unexpectedly large veterinary bill, it allows regular budgeting, which is especially important for older pet owners, many of whom live on fixed incomes.

Clients pay for services in full and then submit the claim directly to the provider for reimbursement. The benefits for veterinarians are that they assume no risk, they are paid when services are rendered, and they usually do not have to handle paperwork.

Companies offering pet health insurance include

- Veterinary Pet Insurance, or VPI (vets.petinsurance.com, 866-Vet-4VPI-for veterinarians and staff 899-4VPI; petinsurance.com or 1-800-USA PETS for clients)
- PetHealth Inc. (petcareinsurance.com; 866-275-PETS)
- The Hartville Group (petshealthplan.com; 800-807-6724)
- The Insurance Corporation of Hannover (www.pethealthinsure.com; 800-Pet Sure)
- PetPartners Inc. (www.petpartnersinc.com; 866-725-2747)
- Petplan (petplan-usa.com; 866-GO PET PLAN)

Again, before buying insurance, it is important for pet owners to read the fine print. Some plans cover only 12 months of care. After that, ongoing conditions are classified as pre-existing and are not subject to coverage. Lifetime-limit policies cover medical expenses up to a given amount; covered-for-life plans cover all the pet's conditions, provided the client remains in good payment standing.

The conditions covered vary as well. At the time of this article's publication, only plans offered by Petplan and PetHealth Inc. cover congenital and hereditary health problems. Preventive care coverage varies among providers, as do benefit schedules that determine payout amounts. Figure out which program you want to recommend and encourage clients to research plans that best suit their individual needs. One size does not fit all.

Benevolent and Hardship Grants

Pets provide companionship for older adults, the disabled, and many others who survive on fixed incomes. Often these loving owners must balance the cost of pet care against the many demands on their pocketbooks. Temporary financial hardship can cause otherwise attentive pet owners to avoid getting help for their sick or injured pets. Likewise, you want to encourage those Good Samaritans who have rescued abandoned animals, but you cannot always expect them to assume the cost for care.

These and other scenarios happen every day, and too often pets go without essential medical care simply because well-intentioned people cannot afford it. Veterinarians on the whole have huge hearts and generously offer pro bono services regularly. At the same time, the practice owner knows it is essential to collect fees that at least offset operating costs. For many veterinarians, compromised treatment is often the only other option they can find.

One solution is a benevolent fund to help cover financial hardship or Good Samaritan cases. There are many approaches for this option. For example, the practice may raise funds through some kind of program (eg, soliciting client donations, offering a grooming day when groomers donate their services to raise money). Many practices establish tribute funds, in which clients send memorial donations to the practice's charitable fund and designate these donations for hardship cases. Other practices elect to set aside a certain percentage of revenues each month specifically for this purpose. A handful of charitable organizations also can help offset such cases, but these programs usually serve limited geographic areas.

Regional or personal funds are not always available. A new program from the AAHA Foundation, called the AAHA Helping Pets Fund, has emerged as part of the solution.

In 2003 the trustees of the AAHA Foundation began to study the idea of offering a nationwide benevolent fund. The AAHA Foundation based its program on the Farley Foundation, a benevolent fund operated by the Ontario Veterinary Medical Association. Launched in 2002, the Farley Foundation provides member practices grants to cover nonelective medical procedures for qualifying clients. Pet owners who participate in Canadian government programs for low-income seniors and disabled persons can apply. Any animal species that provides human companionship is considered. In its first year, the Farley Foundation awarded about 100 grants ranging from $300 to $400.

The AAHA Foundation established its own benevolent fund with $232,000 and began accepting applications on April 1, 2005. Practices can submit an application and documentation through fax, e-mail, or traditional mail.

Grants are based on eligibility rules established by the trustees and are awarded only to AAHA-accredited hospitals. Veterinarians may apply for funding to support cases that meet certain client, treatment, and patient criteria. To be eligible, a case must fit into one of two categories: financial hardship or Good Samaritan.

The Fund awards these grants for nonelective or emergency procedures for sick or injured pets. Routine physical examinations, vaccinations, general dental care, and spays and neuters are not eligible unless the procedure is essential to the animal's continued health.

Documented financial hardship
To prove financial hardship, applying clients must provide documentation in one of two ways.

Pet owners receiving government assistance for low-income individuals or families are eligible. In these cases, documentation of current participation in at least one of the following government assistance programs is submitted with a grant application.

In the United States:

- Food Stamp Program
- Unemployment Insurance
- Supplemental Security Income
- Temporary Assistance for Needy Families
- Medicaid

In Canada:

- Guaranteed Income Supplement
- Old Age Security Allowance
- Old Age Security Allowance for the Survivor
- National Child Benefit Supplement
- Employment Insurance

Temporary financial hardship
In rare circumstances, pet owners experiencing temporary financial hardship may be eligible. In these cases, a letter or e-mail signed or authorized by the veterinarian describing circumstances causing the financial hardship is submitted with a grant application. Third-party supporting documentation is also required. Veterinarians can also apply for financial grants to assist with those Good Samaritan cases in which the owner is not found simply by submitting a letter with a grant application.

For veterinary practices, funding is limited to $500 each calendar year for financial hardship cases and $200 each calendar year for Good Samaritan cases. Practices may submit multiple applications to reach the annual funding limit for each client eligibility category. Each pet and family is limited to $500 during a calendar year. Pet owners may submit multiple applications until they reach the annual funding limit.

Recognizing that treatment decisions often hinge on funding availability, Foundation trustees have adopted a same-day response policy whenever possible, particularly for financial hardship and Good Samaritan cases. The Fund notifies the practice the day a completed application is received, or the next business day if the application is received after office hours. Temporary financial hardship cases usually receive multiple reviews before trustees make their decision. In these cases, the Fund tries to notify applicants within 1 month.

After approval and treatment, grant recipients must submit a detailed invoice to the Fund by fax or regular mail showing required treatment and fees. The Fund then makes the grant payment directly to the veterinary practice, paying in full those invoices that do not exceed established limits and the annual limit in cases that do exceed the limit. Clients do not receive any payments.

There is one caveat: the AAHA Fund requires complete grant application and necessary paperwork. In emergency situations, it is not always feasible to gather such information. Also, the Fund does not accept grant applications for treatments occurring more than 2 weeks before submission. To learn more about fund-raising activities, visit www.aahahelpingpets.org or call toll-free 866-4 HELPETS.

PUT IT ON THE LINE

All hospitals should ask clients up front how they want to handle their financial obligation. The initial visit is the perfect time to discuss pet insurance and financed client payment plans. Have clients apply that day. Remember, you are in the business of offering medical services to clients in need. You are not a loan or charitable institution. By helping educate clients about their financing options, you can remove yourself from the money equation and concentrate on providing what only you can offer: skilled veterinary care.

SUMMARY

Rising veterinary costs can keep some people from accepting necessary medical care for their pets. Viable alternative financing options exist.

For a small fee, third-party finance companies offer clients no-interest or low-interest loans for clients. Practices pay a set-up fee and percentage of loans. Although popular in Europe, pet insurance is still underused in the United States. Coverage plans vary. Benevolent funds, financed though donations to individual practices and some regional organizations, can help cover client hardship and Good Samaritan cases. The AAHA recently introduced a nationwide fund for AAHA-accredited hospitals.

Each alternative comes with its own pros and cons. Practice owners will want to study the offerings carefully to find the best match for their practice and clients.

References

[1] American Pet Products Manufacturers Association; 2004. Available at: http://www. appma.org.

[2] PetPlan USA; 2005. Available at: http://www.petplan-usa.com.

[3] American Pet Products Manufacturers Association; 2000. Available at: http://www. appma.org.

[4] Texas A & M College of Veterinary Medicine. Available at: http://www.cvm.tamu.edu/ oncology/faq/questions/incide01.html.

[5] Veterinary Pet Insurance; 2003. Available at: http://www.petinsurance.com.

[6] National Commission of Veterinary Economic Issues; 2004. Available at: http:// www.ncvei.org.

[7] Brakke Consulting Inc; 2004. Available at: http://www.brakkeconsulting.com.

[8] The path to high quality care. American Animal Hospitals Association; 2003. Available at: http://www.aahanet.org.

[9] Datamonitor report. UK Pet Insurance; 2004. Available at: http://www.datamonitor.com/ ~6117aea910da4b48a8e12d34018f9943~/industries/research/?pid=DMFS1722& type=Report.

[10] The US market for pet health insurance. Packaged Facts; 2003. Available at: http:// www.packagedfacts.com/category/-,-/124.html.

[11] US pet health industry overview. PetPlan USA; 2005. Available at: http://www. petplan-usa.com.

Vet Clin Small Anim 36 (2006) 419–436

VETERINARY CLINICS
SMALL ANIMAL PRACTICE

ELSEVIER
SAUNDERS

Compliance: Crafting Quality Care

Charles J. Wayner, DVM[a],*,
Marsha L. Heinke, DVM, EA, CPA, CVPM[b]

[a]Global Veterinary Practice Health[SM], Hill's Pet Nutrition, Inc., 400 SW Eighth Avenue, Topeka, KS 66603-3945, USA
[b]Marsha L. Heinke, CPA, Inc., 934 Main Street, Grafton, OH 44044, USA

T he word "compliance" has many connotations. In veterinary medicine, compliance traditionally means one of two things:

1. The activities associated with knowing and following laws, regulations, and professional codes or guidelines
2. The degree of client adherence to doctor recommendations and prescribed treatment protocols

Without the veterinary professional's deeper understanding, the latter meaning can be inherently dangerous. Veterinarians may directly or indirectly criticize clients for treatment or preventative health care failures because of perceived less-than-optimal client compliance with recommendations. Instead, veterinary professionals should question whether recommendations were truly made and, if they were, whether they were received, understood, appreciated, and agreed to by the client. Blaming noncompliance solely on the client is an abdication of the veterinary profession's obligation to communicate effectively on behalf of the patient's best interest.

This article challenges the veterinary practitioner and veterinary health care team to recognize and embrace the nuanced aspects of compliance; that is, the

Hill's Pet Nutrition, Inc. funded a $1 million educational grant and other support to the American Animal Hospital Association (AAHA) to sponsor an in-depth study of United States veterinary practices, subsequently known as the 2002 AAHA Compliance Study. The study resulted in AAHA's publication of *The Path to Quality Care: Practical Tips for Improving Compliance,* also subsidized by Hill's Pet Nutrition, Inc. As an employee of Hill's Pet Nutrition, Dr. Wayner was peripherally involved with the study project and subsequently participated in symposia and conference lectures propagating the study's findings and conclusions.

In 2004, Hill's Pet Nutrition funded an additional AAHA project to further knowledge and understanding of veterinary practice protocols and systems that drive superior patient health care through improved compliance. Using grant monies, AAHA engaged Marsha L. Heinke, CPA, Inc. to coordinate, conduct, and report on the project, which included a 2-day focus group of experts to present, compile, and summarize in detail best practices for compliance. Dr. Wayner was one of the 27 Summit attendees.

Financial calculations and contributions were made by Mr. Fritz Wood, CPA, CFP, as a contracted consultant for Hill's Pet Nutrition, Inc.

*Corresponding author. Global Veterinary Practice Health[SM], Hill's Pet Nutrition, Inc., P.O. Box 148, Topeka, KS 66603. *E-mail address:* Chuck_Wayner@hillspet.com (C.J. Wayner).

internal practice systems, protocols, and beliefs that enhance the probability of the best possible veterinary care. Veterinary care occurs not during a single appointment but throughout the patient's life. If, on average, a patient visits the practice twice a year for 30 minutes each visit, that time represents only 0.01% of the year (1 hour divided by 8760 hours in a year). With such limited patient-contact time, the veterinary health care team must firmly establish effective techniques for carrying through on the patient care they advocate as best.

The essence of compliance is crafting quality care. For the reader to understand better the concept's medical and financial importance, this article exposes old paradigms, references insightful data, quantifies opportunities, and encourages change. Crafting quality care (ie, compliance) is in the best interest of the patients, clients, practice, and profession. Compliance is about practicing better medicine, with resultant better business operations that further enhance the delivery of superior medicine.

COMPLIANCE DEFINED

Practicing high-quality veterinary medicine requires proper communication skills and an environment conducive to communicating effectively. To communicate and convey new concepts of veterinary medical practice compliance accurately, commonly accepted terminology must be established.

The human medical field uses the following words for discussing doctor–patient interactions [1]:

Adherence: the extent to which a patient continues an agreed-upon mode of treatment without close supervision

Concordance: a negotiated, shared agreement between clinician and patient concerning treatment regimen(s), outcomes, and behaviors

Protocol: a precise and detailed plan for the study of a biomedical problem for a regimen of therapy

Compliance: the consistency and accuracy with which a patient follows the regimen prescribed by a physician or other health care professionals

Of these terms, compliance best conveys the critical importance of communication for achieving optimal patient care through the twin goals of continuity and consistency. Compliance becomes the centerpiece for fulfilling the veterinary profession's obligation to advocate on behalf of the pet's best interest.

In veterinary medicine, the physician's definition of compliance can be adapted to "the consistency and accuracy with which the client follows the patient-care regimen recommended by the veterinarian." The 2002 American Animal Hospital Association (AAHA) landmark Compliance Study of Veterinary Practices, funded through an educational grant by Hill's Pet Nutrition, Inc., resulted in an even more succinct definition that resonates particularly well with veterinary health care team members: "the pet receives the care (products and services) the veterinarian believes is best for the pet" [2].

If advocating best care for the patient is indeed the essence of practicing veterinary medicine, all members of the profession need to appreciate the benefits of communicating effectively and to understand the ramifications of not communicating well. Compliance is a quality-of-care issue [2] and, as such, should be competently and consistently demonstrated through concern with conviction. Strengthening compliance mandates a practice culture of collaboration, continual learning, systematic application of procedures and protocols, and accurate means of measurement. Measurement tools, such as charts, graphs, computerized database analysis, and reports, help validate improvement.

COMPLIANCE AS A PROCESS

Compliance encompasses virtually every aspect of veterinary practice activity and is dependent on effective communication of recommendations, resulting in informed client acceptance and efficient follow-through for patient care.

Because of the wide scope of compliance and its enormous ramifications on patient care, it is helpful to appreciate the compliance continuum. The AAHA Compliance Study devised an acronym, "CRAFT," to help veterinarian professionals remember the major activities of the compliance cycle as a formula (analogous to, for example, the acronym for learning the major biochemical reactions of the Krebs cycle) [2].

$$\text{Compliance (C)} = \text{Recommendation (R)} + \text{Acceptance (A)} + \text{Follow-through (FT)}$$

Subsequent phases in a cycle cannot take place until the necessary previous processes have occurred. Veterinarians and veterinary health care teams practice their craft every day, so the CRAFT acronym becomes an appropriate framework for prudent practice processes.

Through more comprehensive understanding and implementation of compliance concepts, the veterinary profession can enjoy significant productivity for the benefit of all involved. A 2004 Compliance Summit highlighted a universal theme: compliance must be embraced across the profession's spectrum of activity, from veterinary schools and teaching hospitals through specialists in private practice [3].

Communication

The CRAFT formula can be further distilled to

$$\text{Compliance} = \text{Communication}$$

Communication systems are the prime underpinnings of optimal patient care in any venue. Communication is effective when it creates an emotional connection. The appropriate use of inflection, tone, environment, written instructions, models, and examples enables successful transfer of intended meaning. The effective transfer of meaning involves several separate components: sending > receiving > processing > understanding.

Recommendation

A recommendation is a clear, concise, understandable message delivered regarding the health care team's belief concerning the best action steps for patient health.

Acceptance

Acceptance means that the client receives and understands the intended recommendation, resulting in agreement and informed consent for explicitly defined care for the patient.

Follow-through

The practice's systems, procedures, processes, and protocols result in concise communication to and from all employees concerning the precise care the patient is to receive. Authorized by the informed client, the care parameters (products and services) are reinforced and reaffirmed by competent health care team members. Communicated information includes initial care and the critically important home care, rechecks, revisits, and prescription and product refills. Further recommendations are communicated as needed.

Compliance in care is a continuum, not a conclusion. Communication is the continuum's cornerstone.

COMPLACENCY ABOUT COMPLIANCE

Historically, compliance was often attributed to or blamed on the client. Did the client do what the veterinarian and health care team recommended? If so, client compliance was said to have occurred. If the client did not do something that purportedly was recommended, the client was alleged to be noncompliant.

For many, the thought process ended there, with little reflection on how, or even why, the patient–owner–veterinarian interaction could be more beneficial and productive. The AAHA study provided data and evidence that alleged client-compliance failures are commonly and directly attributable to communication lapses by the veterinary health care team.

When asked, 78% of veterinarians indicated that they were satisfied with the level of compliance in their practices. The major reason for this satisfaction is that almost no one actually measured compliance. Rather, they assumed high rates of compliance and estimated percentages of compliance. Virtually all veterinarians guessed that their compliance rates were much higher than they really were [2]. Not measuring existing compliance is the largest single barrier to achieving higher compliance [2].

Client surveys indicated that nearly 60% agreed that their veterinarian did not always make clear the importance of health care recommendations [2]. For example, client survey questions about senior care revealed that only 30% of older pets had received diagnostic screenings. The remaining 70% responded they had "never heard of it," "didn't know I should do it," or "my veterinarian never recommended or suggested it" [2]. Although veterinarians and health care team members often believe they have made recommendations, client perception is often just the opposite. The findings indicate that effective communication (connecting) had not occurred.

Do you help clients to be more compliant, by allowing them to make informed buying decisions, or do you avoid the issue, leaving them confused and therefore unable to act on your suggestions?

THE COMPELLING CASE FOR CRAFTING COMPLIANCE

One definition of "care" is "watchful attention." One definition of "client" is "a dependent." Coupling the definitions shows the new concept of compliance as an extremely powerful call to action for the veterinary profession.

Compliance is all about "caring about care," (a theme in the veterinary profession that will never go out of style) [4]. The 'C' which stands for Compliance in the "CRAFT" acronym could be also stand for Care, Conviction, Concern, Communication, Cooperation, Compassion, Crusade, Customization, Continuity, Convenience, and Client-Centric!

Furthermore, think about the R in the acronym "CRAFT," which stands for Recommendation. Veterinarians communicate effective, professional, and ethical guidance to their clients in the form of recommendations. The confident and competent veterinary health care team communicates and reinforces recommendations. Highly effective teams commonly use scripted language for powerful dialogue and increased understanding, such as "Your pet needs and deserves x, y, and z" [5].

Acceptance (the 'A' in "CRAFT") implies informed client consent and all the mandatory verbal and written communications, both legally and ethically prescribed, required to obtain the client's agreement and approval.

Follow-through (the 'FT' in "CRAFT") by the veterinary health care team helps ensure exact and complete client-authorized patient care, in accordance with the practice's standards, including all home-care instructions, reminders, recalls, and recheck appointments. Technology can provide many more options for effective client follow-up communication, and most clients are receptive and appreciative of such efforts.

Early adopters of compliance-improvement programs in veterinary practice have recognized significant challenges in design, implementation, and measurement. To address these challenges the American Animal Hospital Association sponsored a Compliance Summit in June 2004. A prime goal was to identify effective, replicable tools, work processes, and systems that would result in improved patient care, increases in revenue and transactions, and greater productivity by the veterinary health care team. To solicit useful information and key experience, participants were asked about best practices. The project designers defined "best practices" as a term describing behaviors, leadership characteristics, protocols, and procedures that yield a desired outcome, in this case consistent, quality care [3].

Summit participants had a history of having implemented protocols to address measured compliance gaps in their own practices or of having consulting with practices implementing such protocols. Practices should conduct this type of discovery process with their teams to develop and use concepts that best fit the practices' culture [3]. Using a lessons-learned approach, the Summit participants identified the following best practices as possible ways to elevate compliance:

- Design/refine/reaffirm the practice's mission statement, the conscience of the practice.
- Create a practice culture that inspires compliance.
- "Diagnose before you prescribe": review medical records to realize the opportunities [2].
- Focus on and master one area of compliance at a time.
- Use agreed-upon written protocols, procedures, and standards.
- Make extensive use of reminders and call backs (telephone or e-mail).
- Document effective scripts, with careful use of language to deliver the right message.
- Use forms and checklists to ensure consistent recommendations by all members of the health care team.
- Enjoin repetitive training, skill set development and role-playing.
- Use judicious reward systems to recognize goal accomplishment.
- Emphasize care issues rather than money or practice financial issues.
- Systematically conduct regular medical record reviews and audits.
- Pre-chart medical records in advance of scheduled client appointments.
- Use patient chart stickers to enable consistent recommendations.
- Systematically measure progress and promptly share results with the entire health care team.
- Designate a full- or part-time employee to review charts and function as a patient advocate.
- Institute job titles and descriptions for compliance-related responsibilities (eg, Patient Advocate, Medical Standards Officer, Client Liaison, or Patient Care Coordinator).
- Implement practice management software options for linked-invoice messages.
- Use computer generated recommendation codes.
- Use computer management software as much as possible to track results.

During the AAHA Compliance Summit, participants revealed some of their methods for gaining total health team commitment to compliance concepts [3]. The following beneficial insights are worthy of consideration:

Develop and promote a practice culture and philosophy in concert with the health care team and in concrete terms. Quality of care and compliance are professional responsibilities. Quality of care constitutes a long-term plan for practice and patient health that emphasizes prevention rather than intervention.

Prevention philosophy centers in plans that consider the entire patient over its entire life expectancy rather than the myopic view of each medical problem as it evolves. For practice compliance programs to accomplish quality-of-care goals successfully, every person on the practice team must be engaged.

Stoking the passion for compliance throughout the entire team requires positive, tangible practice leadership. Think through the compliance plan details, be well prepared, and have specific answers ready for anticipated questions. Instill and reinforce confidence in the team that championing compliance is continually relevant [6].

Understand what motivates employee subsets. Discuss how compliance drives the technical application of quality medicine to spark doctor enthusiasm. For the health care team, lead discussions about how compliance makes for better patient care. To gain commitment from reception personnel, emphasize how compliance relates to the family-pet-veterinary team bond. To gain agreement from management, emphasize how improved compliance directly leads to better business and productivity [3].

THE COMPLIANCE CONTINUUM

Effective compliance systems for quality care require consistency in transitioning primary patient responsibilities and communications from one team member to another within the practice as well as to external team members. The practice's health care team must coordinate effective communication and tasks with clients and client families and, as necessary, with specialists, reference laboratories, vendors, and product and service representatives.

Communication never stops, and compliance is not an endpoint (the client did or did not do something) but rather a continuum. Each step in the following compliance continuum presents the health care team with opportunities to influence pet care positively [7]:

> A pet worth having →
> A thorough examination worth conducting →
> A diagnosis (regarding wellness or disease management) worth making →
> Protocols worth advocating →
> Effective recommendations (with conviction) worth communicating →
> Products and services worth providing →
> Health care team skills worth demonstrating →
> Client acceptance worth encouraging →
> Benefits worth reiterating/reinforcing →
> Proper client understanding/use worth checking →
> Continued use/care worth stressing →
> Rechecks/return visits, repurchases worth scheduling →
> Great medicine worth practicing →
> Being an advocate for the patient's best interest

Consider this simplified process for a patient wellness visit:

- The client receives a reminder or remembers it is time for the pet's checkup.
- The client telephones the practice to set up an appointment for a checkup.
- The receptionist reviews the appointment book and schedules a physical examination.
- The client brings the pet to practice for appointment.
- The receptionist checks in the client and patient.
- The patient is weighed.

- The designated employee escorts the client and patient to an examination room.
- The veterinarian performs the patient physical examination.
- The examination information is recorded in patient record.
- The veterinarian gives the client verbal recommendations.
- The client decides to purchase recommended products or services at that time, to schedule another visit, or think about some of the mentioned products or services for future purchase.
- The client exits to the reception area to pay for products or services bought/performed that day.
- The receptionist files a reminder for the patient's next physical examination.
- The client receives some sort of reminder at some point in the future.

A practice using this work process abdicates to the client the responsibility for nearly all aspects of patient care. Compliance depends on the client's action; the client either does or does not comply.

Veterinary practice administrators should eagerly and aggressively rally to change this paradigm. The compliance continuum shows many opportunities to enhance the veterinary-practice experience for all involved. The following discussion indicates the points at which the veterinary health care team can proactively enhance compliance.

CONTINUITY OF CARE

When a client presents a pet to a veterinary practice for care, the client implicitly (if not explicitly) says, "At this moment, my pet's health is a priority to me." The health care team creates value for the client by making the patient, at that moment, the team's priority, too. Value results from real or perceived benefits greater than the client's costs of time and money. How can that value best be created, especially in a busy practice?

Positive influence points are those moments in the practice–client interaction at which the health care team can create value as well as proactively direct high-quality care and compliance. The goal is to provide what the client wants (and values), which happens to be congruent with the health care team's delivering the care the patient needs and deserves.

When the practice purposefully orchestrates what happens during each positive influence point, the health care team adds substantial value to the client's experience and increases compliance with the practice's standards of care. Health care teams can practice the following exercise (Box 1) during team meetings. With repeated practice, the exercise results in greater team member synergy and productivity.

Use the previous wellness visit process example as an exercise template. The following suggestions provide insights into possible ways to enhance the client and patient experience.

At the first influence point, the client receives some sort of reminder or remembers that it is time for the pet's checkup. Box 2 lists ways the health care team can positively influence compliance in issuing appointment reminders.

Box 1: Exercise in increasing compliance by adding value at positive influence points

The meeting leader proposes a specific influence point. The team brainstorms creative ways to increase or improve client value. A designated scribe lists the ideas that will later be incorporated in standard operating procedure. The exercise calls on practice personnel either to support or redesign current practice procedures, thereby reinforcing the team's uniform approach. The practice system becomes increasingly defined and ingrained.

The next positive influence point occurs when the client telephones the practice for an appointment. The receptionist reviews the appointment book and schedules a physical examination for the patient. Box 3 lists ways the health care team can positively influence compliance when scheduling an appointment.

The client brings the pet to the practice. The receptionist checks in the client and the patient. The patient is weighed. Box 4 lists the ways the ways the health care team can positively influence compliance during and after check in.

The team member escorts the client and pet to an examination room. Box 5 lists ways the health care team can positively influence compliance during the pre-examination period and examination.

The veterinarian performs patient physical examination. Examination information is documented in the patient's record. The veterinarian makes recommendations. Box 6 lists steps, in addition to the veterinarian's comprehensive physical examination, that can positively influence compliance at this point.

The client purchases some products or services at that time, schedules another visit, or defers decisions to consider some of the mentioned products

---

Box 2: How the health care team can positively influence compliance in issuing appointment reminders

In sending appointment reminders, the health care team can positively influence compliance by

• Sending or calling a reminder far enough in advance of the time for the actual examination so the client can plan accordingly

• Letting the client know the reminder will be made, so the client can rely on you; emphasize the importance of such a visit

• Asking the client about the preferred mode of reminder contact

• Designing and scripting reminders for impact, whether by mail, e-mail or telephone

• Being specific about the pet's individual needs, as predefined through current practice standards (proper pet nutrition, parasite control, oral health, weight management, and other concerns)

Box 3: How the health care team can positively influence compliance when scheduling an appointment

- Be courteous and attentive on the phone; use the client's and pet's names and know how to pronounce them correctly.
- Reference the pet's medical record to identify other care needs in addition to the examination; mentioning possible needs, based on the practice's predetermined care standards.
- Identify a date and time convenient for the client.
- Inquire about other pets in the household.
- Inform the client you will telephone the day before, as a courtesy reminder.
- Suggest the client (including family members) prepare written questions in advance to ask during the appointment.
- Confidently describe key health issues the team will reinforce during the visit.
- Verify pertinent client contact and patient information.
- Confirm the client knows the practice location and advise of potential traffic problems such as road construction information.
- Twenty-four hours before the appointment provide telephone confirmation and remind the client to prepare questions to ask of the veterinarian and health care team.

or services. The client proceeds to the reception area and pays for products or services bought/performed that day. Box 7 describes some of the ways the health care team can positively influence compliance as the office visit ends.

Box 4: How the health care can team positively influence compliance during and after check in

- Prepare the patient record a day in advance of the appointment.
- Telephone the client before the appointment time, if necessary, to inform her of any delays/emergencies.
- Maintain an orderly, pleasant, and odor-free reception area.
- Welcome the client and pet by name.
- Verify client contact data.
- Refer to the medical record and note any cued points to discuss.
- Weigh the pet and record weight. Compare the weight with the patient's weight history.
- Verify the diet and record it in the medical record.
- Minimize waiting time.
- Maximize personalized client contact time through orchestrated pairing of the team members with the client.

Box 5: How the health care team can positively influence compliance before and during the examination

- Escort the client and pet, assisting where appropriate.
- Apprise the client about which team members will next enter the examination room (eg, technician, veterinarian, assistant).
- Use an examination room appropriately sized for the pet and client/family.
- Enthusiastically outline key areas the team wants to reinforce and provide correlating printed documentation.
- Pre-orchestrate which team member asks the client for what information. Do not repetitively ask for the same information except to obtain additional insights or clarification.
- Record any patient information and data to assist the veterinarian's examination and discussions.

GAPS IN COMPLIANCE

In the compliance continuum, any missed opportunities are called gaps. For example, the number of active canine patients will be larger than the number of active canine patients who are currently receiving medication for heartworm prevention. The difference between the two statistics is a measure of compliance. If the practice standards state all canine patients should be medicated with heartworm preventative, the gap suggests less-than-optimal care.

Practice systems, protocols, and persistent development of employee skills establish consistent, replicable steps in the compliance continuum. Compliance

Box 6: Further ways the health care team can positively influence compliance during and after the physical examination

- Thoroughly review the patient's record, noting previous recommendations, treatments, and client refusals or deferrals. What were the reasons for recommendations, treatments, and, if any, refusals?
- Review and discuss weight history.
- Complete the patient examination report card, noting current observations (body condition score, periodontal grade, attitude, and so forth), concerns and kudos, and specific recommendations.
- Review all conclusions with the client, using effective communication techniques. Convey findings with confidence, competence, enthusiasm, care, and patience. Support verbal communication with practiced body language, visual aids, and other materials that enhance the connection with the client for optimal transmittal of information.
- Reinforce the key health issues consistent with prior targeted topics.
- Create the best possible examination room ambiance to optimize communications between client and the medical team. Minimize distractions to the extent possible.

Box 7: How the health care team can positively influence compliance at the end of the office visit

- At this moment, the pet is the client's top priority. Assert that the pet is your priority at that moment, too.

- Make clear and succinct recommendations based on all dialogue and procedures to that point and dictated by practice standards. Do not give the client a menu of suggestions and options.

- Positively affirm the importance of the recommendations. Do not make recommendations off-handedly. Give the client a clear understanding of what steps should be taken next.

- If the client does not take action, do not immediately assume that the client is not concerned about the pet. The problem, (therefore the opportunity) may not be one of client noncompliance but rather one of client confusion.

- Do not suggest that the health care team should be aggressive in trying to get the pet owner to agree to something the client does not feel comfortable doing or authorizing. At the same time, do not put all the blame on the client. Clearly communicate best recommendations.

- To achieve application (client use of the practice's products and services), you must first achieve understanding through excellent communication (the successful transfer of intended meaning [ie, sending > receiving > processing > understanding]).

- You have an obligation to help the client comply by honing your own compliance skills. Maximize the possibility that the pet receives the practice's top standard of quality care.

- Schedule follow-up communication if the client elects to postpone a procedure or the purchase of a product.

- Practice scripted responses to use when a client defers by stating the need to discuss things with other family members. Such deferrals are often responsible responses in the client's situation, which may not be fully known to you.

- Approach scheduled rechecks, new appointments, and product refills in the same, consistent manner.

ratios equal the patient numbers current with predetermined practice standards of care as compared with all patients in that practice demographic. The following list identifies points in a practice's workflow at which best practices can improve compliance ratios, in this example, for a product:

Veterinarian examines patient **GAP** Condition(s) identified
Condition(s) identified **GAP** Condition(s) documented
Condition(s) documented **GAP** Condition(s) communicated
Condition(s) communicated **GAP** Recommendations made
Recommendations made **GAP** Client may/may not accept
If client does not accept **GAP** Document and revisit/remind
If client agrees **GAP** Communicate proper use
Communicate proper use **GAP** Client purchase
Client purchase **GAP** Client use

Client use **GAP** Team reinforcement (telephone call or other follow-up)
Team reinforcement **GAP** Client feedback
Client feedback **GAP** Health care team reiteration
Health care team reiteration **GAP** Client's continual use
Client's continual use **GAP** Client revisits/repurchases
Client revisits/repurchases **GAP** Better patient care
Better patient care **GAP** Enhanced team productivity

ENHANCED TEAM PRODUCTIVITY LEADS TO GREAT MEDICINE/GREAT BUSINESS

With every process, practice personnel have opportunities to close the gap (to move on to the next step in the continuum) or to widen the gap (in effect, impairing practice goals for achieving improved quality of care and all of its positive economic attributes). Compliance is a multifaceted process that relies on a cascade of events to achieve a decisive, favorable situation in the pet's best interest. The earlier that a breakdown occurs in the process, the more adverse are the effects on achieving practice goals.

CLARIFYING CONCERNS

Every member of the health care team plays an important role in clarifying concerns. By increasing the client's understanding about veterinary recommendations and through the health care team's reinforcing clarifications, compliance ratios increase.

The AAHA Compliance Study suggested that clients are often confused or mistaken about patient care recommendations. A prime goal of employee training is developing and enhancing communication skills. Doctors and others on the health care team may assume they have competently informed the client about what to do and why; however, the team often does not confirm with the client whether true understanding occurred.

Clients become confused when members of the health care team use language that is too medically based, offer a variety of choices, or make vague, passive comments such as "her teeth need attention." All such communication errors detract from the ability to deliver high-caliber care.

Passive, indirect language and vague statements are open to a wide variety of interpretation. Do not assume clients or coworkers know precisely what you mean or how to do something you direct. Clarify your statements and the person's understanding by probing with a question such as, "Could you describe for me in your own words what I've just presented, so I can determine whether I've communicated effectively?"

You should also affirm you understand what the other person has tried to communicate to you: "Let me make sure I understand what you are saying. What I hear you saying is ... Is my understanding correct"? In discussions, check understandings from time to time in this manner to help maximize effective communications.

Remember your body language may unwittingly convey a message that is completely opposite to the meaning of the words. Studies show that body language greatly affects communication. Body language may substantially override verbal communication, to the point that observed facial expressions and postures leave much more powerful memories than the spoken word.

Teach everyone on the health care team to recognize and know what non-verbal messages may subliminally convey, including, for example, clothing styles, fragrances, jewelry, and hairstyles. Role-playing during video recording is a powerful training method. Assure that the spoken word is accompanied by appropriate body language, voice inflection, and sincerity.

Provide visual and printed support material to aid in the communication process. Although such adjunct tools reinforce message and memory, information overload can decrease retention related to recommendations. Do not automatically try to convey every detail. Work at understanding different personality types to realize if and when a person might require more or less information. Realize the importance of modifying your own preferred way of communicating to that based on the client's needs.

Promptly adapt new medical knowledge into easily explained and understandable concepts. Clients and coworkers rely on the clear communications to make informed decisions and take correct action.

COMPLIANCE PAYS OFF

The AAHA Compliance Study provided a clear, simple, and proven process for improving compliance [2]; however, simple does not mean "easy." The process still requires a positively persuasive practice culture. If the entire veterinary health care team commits to the fervent belief that increased compliance means better medicine, then the practice will benefit from better business.

The 2004 American Veterinary Medical Association (AVMA)-Pfizer Business Practices Study conducted by Brakke Consulting, Inc., shows a significant increase in veterinary incomes since 1997 of 41% after inflation [8]. Evidence suggests that the most of that increase came from fee increases. Although fee increases typically were long overdue, continually raising prices without increasing the client-perceived value of the veterinary experience is not the best, most sustainable long-term strategy.

From a pet health and business health perspective, the best strategy targets improved compliance in many aspects of patient care. Relatively few pets actually receive the care the veterinary profession believes best for them. Consider three examples from the AAHA Compliance Study findings. Of the opportunities investigated, the study found these areas to be the most economically viable and, in general, the most achievable after considering various geographic, climatic, and seasonal issues [2]:

- Dental prophylaxis: 29% compliance; 71% noncompliance
- Therapeutic nutrition: 5% compliance; 95% noncompliance
- Senior screenings: 33% compliance; 67% noncompliance

Dental Prophylaxis

According to the AVMA, a typical small-animal veterinarian examines 38 to 43 patients each week [9]. With a patient load of seven patients per day, per doctor, performing one more periodontal prophylaxis procedure each day results in incremental per doctor gross income per year of $76,320 [10]. (The median dental case totals $265 [sum of the fees for the pre-anesthetic examination, complete blood cell count with differential, eight chemistries, 30 minutes of anesthesia, intravenous catheter and placement, intravenous fluids, scaling and polishing, subgingival curettage, fluoride application, electronic monitoring, postoperative pain medication, postoperative antibiotics, and hospitalization] × 288 days [6 d/wk, 48 wk/y] = $76,320.)

The AAHA Compliance Study suggests that 50% of clients who received a recommendation for periodontal therapy followed through with the therapy. Of the remaining 50%, at least half were likely to schedule the procedure and could have complied relatively easily if the practice had followed up on the recommendation [2]. Only a very small percentage of clients (7%) declined dental care for their pet because of cost [2].

Given existing compliance rates, perhaps one or two of the seven patients a doctor sees in one day will have received periodontal therapy within the past year or so, leaving several potential candidates untended. According to Jan Bellows, DVM, DAVDC, DABVP, "Research shows that 80 percent of dogs and 70 percent of cats show signs of gingival disease by the age of three according to the American Veterinary Dental Society" [11]. Disease prevalence and compliance rates indicate that performing one periodontal therapy procedure a day is entirely realistic and feasible in the average practice. The latent demand exists.

This analysis does not account for two other factors that could improve the practice's economic picture:

1. As a result of performing more dental procedures, the practice will be able to provide additional oral care products and services.
2. If improved oral health results in increased longevity, the lifetime contribution of that pet to a practice increases.

Therapeutic Nutrition

Beginning and subsequently sustaining one patient per day on an appropriate plane of therapeutic nutrition results in incremental per doctor gross income per year of $33,013 [12]. This result could occur without seeing any new patients.

Evidence suggests that although pet owners want a specific nutritional recommendation, few receive one. The AAHA Compliance Study suggests that a majority of clients (55%) purchased the recommended food when a therapeutic pet food recommendation was made [2]. Further, the study conveys that only a small percentage of clients (4%) declined therapeutic food because of cost, and "pet owners ... were willing to spend more for a recommended diet if it would help their pets" [2].

Given existing compliance rates, it is likely that none of the seven patients a doctor sees per day are using a therapeutic nutritional product. But among these patients are obese patients and patients that have periodontal disease, gastrointestinal issues, arthritic disease, heart disease, kidney disease, dermatologic conditions, urinary tract problems, and diabetes. Disease prevalence and compliance rates indicate that moving a pet per day to a therapeutic nutritional product is realistic and feasible. The latent demand exists.

This analysis is conservative in that it omits several concepts that could significantly enhance the economics:

1. Sales of products such as therapeutic foods can increase client interactions in a veterinary practice, and these client visits drive sales of ancillary products and services [12]. (The average 40-pound dog consumes 200 pounds of food each year. At a selling price of $1.64 per pound (calculation on file), 200 × $1.64 = $328.00. The average 10-pound cat consumes 50 pounds of food each year. At a selling price of $2.61 per pound (calculation on file), 50 × $2.61 = $130.50. Average for dogs and cats = $229.25 {($328.00 + $130.50)/2}. One dog or cat started on January 1, and another started on December 31; the average of a dog or cat started on June 30 or July 1 = $114.63 ($229.25/2) × 288 days (6 d/wk, 48 wk/y) = $33,013.44 [12].)

2. The calculations do not account for the practice opportunity to encourage whole-life wellness plans for longevity through excellent nutrition for disease prevention.

3. If a sick or diseased pet is consistently fed a practice-dispensed therapeutic food, it may live longer. Increased longevity dramatically increases the lifetime contribution of that pet to the practice.

Senior Screenings

Performing one more senior screening each day results in incremental per doctor gross income per year of $28,080 [10].

According to the AAHA Compliance Study, "When senior screenings were recommended, 70 percent of dog owners and 74 percent of cat owners accepted the recommendation" [2]. Only a small percentage of clients (5%) declined senior screenings because of cost [2].

AAHA data classified 35% of dogs and cats as seniors [2], so two or three of the seven patients seen per doctor per day fit that demographic. Performing one more senior screening each day per veterinarian seems entirely realistic and feasible. The latent demand exists.

This analysis does not account for two other factors that could improve the economic picture:

1. As a result of performing more senior screenings, practices will provide additional relevant products and patient services based on screening results.

2. Addressing existing or possible issues uncovered in the senior screenings result could result in increased longevity for the pet, boosting the lifetime contribution of that pet to a practice.

Summary: The Gross Revenue Per Doctor Per Year
 Dental prophylaxis $76,320
 Therapeutic nutrition $33,013
 Senior screenings $28,080
 Total $137,413

According to the AVMA, a typical small-animal exclusive practitioner generates a gross income of $322,768 [9]. If compliance improves as outlined previously, gross income per doctor per year increases to $460,181, a 43% increase. The examples outlined here represent only a small portion of a practice's potential when implementing compliance-enhancing concepts. Improved compliance is a valid, worthy solution to less-than-optimal patient care and also to poor revenue growth.

A CALL TO ACTION

Systems for continual development and refinement of the veterinary health care team's compliance competencies enhance patient care. Veterinarians can no longer blame clients for the underuse of the veterinary team's skills, talents, knowledge, abilities, products, and services. Although the client makes the final decision as to what the health care team can or cannot do for the patient, the veterinary team is duty bound to communicate consistent recommendations effectively.

Effective communication systems are key to the compliance continuum. Clients depend on appropriate recommendations and reinforcement from competent and confident veterinary health care team members. Thoughtful, contemporary, uniform practice protocols and continual skill-set improvement inspire confidence that permeates the practice atmosphere.

At the beginning of this article, the authors challenged the veterinary health care team to discover and implement internal practice systems, policies, and protocols that enhance the probability of delivering the best possible veterinary care. Certainly, what defines "best possible" may be considered a matter of choice. The spectrum of opinion develops from individuals, specialties, institutions, and organizations, regionally and nationally, and is especially dependent upon the culture of the practice.

In the absence of common definitions and professional guidelines of best practices, standards of care are ill defined and arbitrary. In the legal arena, "standard of care" is a moving target. Comparison with one's peers—what a trier of fact determines as customary and usual—becomes the ruler by which a veterinarian's care is judged.

Measurement becomes the final determinant of whether a practice has effectively crafted high-quality care. Compliance demands measurable goals. Measurable goals are based on standards. Until the veterinary profession as a whole fully embraces agreed-upon standards, veterinary practice directors must design, orchestrate, and adapt internally based standards for their own practices and ensure consistency in the communication of those standards.

Practice and professional leadership truly drives compliance, in all of its veterinary nuances and connotations. Document standards and establish practical systems for measurement and accountability. Craft, orchestrate, and practice compliance-enhancing programs for the sake of the patients, the clients, the health care team, the profession, and yourself. It is often said that people don't care how much you know, until they know how much you care.

Demonstrate your sincerity in crafting quality care through improved compliance.

References

[1] Stedman's online medical dictionary. Available at: http://www.stedmans.com. Accessed August 22, 2005.

[2] The path to high quality care. Practical tips for improving compliance. Denver (CO): American Animal Hospital Association; 2003.

[3] Heinke ML. Learning how to CRAFT quality care. Presented at the American Animal Hospital Association Compliance Summit, Denver, CO, 2004.

[4] Hawn R. Learning how to CRAFT quality care. Presented at the American Animal Hospital Association Compliance Summit, Denver, CO, 2004.

[5] Downing R. Learning how to CRAFT quality care. Presented at the American Animal Hospital Association Compliance Summit, Denver, CO, 2004.

[6] Drake M. Learning how to CRAFT quality care. Presented at the American Animal Hospital Association Compliance Summit, Denver, CO, 2004.

[7] Veterinary Nutritional Advocate on-line curriculum. Available at: http://www.VNA.HillsVet.com. Accessed September 9, 2005.

[8] Looking forward to a prosperous year. Veterinary Economics 2005;Aug:12–6.

[9] Economic report on veterinarians and veterinary practices. Journal of the American Veterinary Medical Association 2005;76:225.

[10] The veterinary fee reference. 4th edition. Denver (CO): American Animal Hospital Association; 2005. p. 283.

[11] Bellows J. Oral healthcare products. DVM Best Practices 2005;Jan:12–5.

[12] KPMG study: revelations on Hill's product profitability. Topeka (KS): Hill's Pet Nutrition, Inc., 2003.

Vet Clin Small Anim 36 (2006) 437–441

VETERINARY CLINICS
SMALL ANIMAL PRACTICE

INDEX

Note: Page numbers of article titles are in **boldface** type.

Changing Your Address?

Make sure your subscription changes too! When you notify us of your new address, you can help make our job easier by including an exact copy of your Clinics label number with your old address (see illustration below.) This number identifies you to our computer system and will speed the processing of your address change. Please be sure this label number accompanies your old address and your corrected address—you can send an old Clinics label with your number on it or just copy it exactly and send it to the address listed below.

We appreciate your help in our attempt to give you continuous coverage. Thank you.

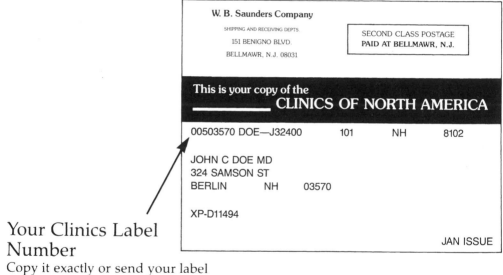

Your Clinics Label Number
Copy it exactly or send your label along with your address to:
W.B. Saunders Company, Customer Service
Orlando, FL 32887-4800
Call Toll Free 1-800-654-2452

Please allow four to six weeks for delivery of new subscriptions and for processing address changes.